The HUNGER HERO DIET

Fast and easy recipe series #3

tinned fish
Vietnamese-style

Kathryn M. James

Copyright © 2023 by Kathryn M James

All Rights Reserved.
No part of this book may be used or reproduced by any means, graphic, electronic, or mechanical, including photocopying, recording, taping, or by any information storage retrieval system without the written permission of the copyright owner, except in the case of brief quotations embodied in critical articles and reviews.

The Working Alliance, Gold Coast, Australia
ISBN 978-0-6455255-8-8

https://kmjameswriter.com/

This edition may contain product information specific to the supermarket shopping experience in Australasia.

Disclaimer

Neither the author nor the publisher can be held liable to any person or entity with respect to any loss or damage caused, or alleged to be caused, directly or indirectly, by the information contained in this work or associated media. As any scientist will affirm, results may vary, so no guarantee is given or implied with regard to information supplied. It is general information only.

It is not the intent of the author to diagnose or prescribe. The intent is only to offer health information to help you cooperate with your medical professionals in your mutual quest for health. In the event you use this information without their approval, you are prescribing for yourself, which is your right, but the publisher and author assume no responsibility. While every precaution has been taken to ensure the information presented herein is accurate, there are many factors beyond the control of the author.

Before starting any diet, you should speak to your doctor. Do not rely on information in this book as an alternative to medical advice. If you have any specific questions about any medical matter, consult your medical practitioner.

All trademarks or brand names mentioned by the author, in this book or elsewhere, remain unreservedly the property of their respective owners, and no claim is made to them, and no endorsement by them is implied or claimed.

Table of Contents

Introduction...11
    How to make rice paper rolls................................. 15
    How to prepare rice noodles.................................. 18
    How to eat the rainbow...22
    How to add flavour... 25

TINNED TUNA... 29

TUNA ROLLS with all the basics................................... 31
    1. Tuna, ginger, avo, Asian slaw................................ 32
    2. Tuna, sambal, kaleslaw.. 33
    3. Tuna, avo, mixed slaw..34
    4. Tuna, chilli, avo, kaleslaw......................................35
    5. Tuna, spicy slaw, onion flakes............................. 36
    6. Tuna, chilli, dill, kaleslaw...................................... 37
    7. Tuna, sambal, Thai mizuna.................................. 38
    8. Tuna, Trident chilli, herbs.....................................39
    9. Tuna, Asian salad slaw..40
    10. Tuna, Sambal, Oakleaf...41
    11. Tuna, Gochujang, lemon thyme....................... 42
    12. Tuna, sambal, mint, fennel.................................43
    13. Tuna, sambal, coleslaw, lime............................. 44
    14. Tuna, avo, beetroot, fennel................................ 45
    15. Tuna, guacamole, kaleslaw.................................46
    16. Tuna, kaleslaw, alfalfa.. 47

17. Tuna, vinegar, jalapenos, Viet mint.................48
18. Tuna, dill, dried onion flakes........................ 49
19. Tuna, Fukujinzuke, pea sprouts...................50
20. Tuna, Fukujinzuke, shallots, mint................ 52
21. Tuna, Fukujinsuke, coriander, fennel...........53
22. Tuna, sambal, Viet mint................................ 54
23. Tuna, Trident, kaleslaw, Oakleaf................. 55
24. Tuna, chilli, Viet mint, fennel...................... 56
25. Tuna, chilli, lime, coriander......................... 57
26. Tuna, spicy kaleslaw, coriander...................58
27. Tuna, jalapenos, kaleslaw, alfalfa................ 59
28. Tuna, Trident, coleslaw................................ 60
29. Tuna, green avo salad, vinegar.................... 61
30. Tuna, green avo salad, fennel......................62

TUNA ROLLS without yoghurt............................... 63

31. Tuna, spicy Thai mizuna, sambal................ 64
32. Tuna, chilli, mizuna, Caesar........................ 65
33. Tuna, kale, herbs, Chang's...........................66
34. Tuna, spicy vinegar, Viet mint..................... 67
35. Tuna, lime, sambal, Thai mizuna.................68
36. Tuna, pickled onion, coriander.................... 69
37. Tuna, onion, alfalfa, Chang's.......................70
38. Tuna, jalapenos, coleslaw, fennel.................71
39. Tuna, baby leaf, Trident, Thai basil............. 72

40. Tuna, silverbeet, pineapple, lemon......73
41. Tuna, fennel root, bean sprouts...... 74
42. Tuna, fennel root, lime, coriander......75
43. Tuna, sauerkraut, kale, beets...... 76
44. Tuna, tahini, jalapenos, mint...... 77

TUNA ROLLS without avocado......78

45. Tuna, Viet mint, mixed slaw......79
46. Tuna, Thai mizuna, herbs...... 80
47. Tuna, kale, alfalfa...... 81
48. Tuna, Trident, onion, dill...... 82
49. Tuna, chilli, onion, mixed slaw...... 83
50. Tuna, kaleslaw, Chang's sauce......84
51. Tuna, grilled capsicum, pineapple...... 85
52. Tuna, tahini, beetroot, jalapenos...... 86

TUNA ROLLS with nori...... 88

53. Tuna, nori, sambal, avo, fennel...... 89
54. Tuna, nori, ginger, dill......90
55. Tuna, nori, chilli, onion flakes...... 91
56. Tuna, nori, Viet mint, fennel......93
57. Tuna, nori, basil, fennel...... 94
58. Tuna, nori, kaleslaw......95
59. Tuna, nori, Trident, kaleslaw......96
60. Tuna, nori, lime, mint...... 97
61. Tuna, nori, avo, kaleslaw...... 98

62. Tuna, nori, grilled capsicum, bean sprouts........99
63. Tuna, nori, grilled capsicum, coriander...........101
64. Tuna, nori, chilli, alfalfa............................102

TUNA ROLLS with a hint of Mediterranean.........103

65. Tuna, balsamic, baby leaves.......................104
66. Tuna, balsamic, dill, alfalfa.........................105
67. Tuna, balsamic, mizuna, dill.......................106
68. Tuna, balsamic, mizuna, onion flakes..........107
69. Tuna, balsamic, onion, lime........................108
70. Tuna, balsamic, dill, tartare sauce...............109
71. Tuna, balsamic, coleslaw, alfalfa.................110
72. Tuna, balsamic, Gochujang, lettuce............111
73. Tuna, kalamata, chilli, basil........................112
74. Tuna, tomato, mizuna, tartare sauce...........113

TUNA SALAD BOWLS..................................114

75. Tuna, mizuna salad, onion flakes...............116
76. Spicy tuna, tomato, dill salad....................117
77. Spicy tuna, yoghurt salad.........................118
78. Tuna, pineapple, crunchy noodle salad......119
79. Tuna and warm asparagus salad...............120
80. Tuna, Caesar rainbow salad......................121
81. Italian tuna, balsamic, olive salad..............122
82. Italian tuna, olive, tomato salad................123
83. Spicy Italian tuna, basil salad....................124

84. Italian tuna, tomato, artichoke salad................ 125

85. The Traveller, tuna, noodle salad...................... 126

86. Tuna, coleslaw, noodle salad............................. 127

87. Tonkatsu tuna with warm noodle salad........... 128

TINNED TUNA in SOUPS.. 129

88. Indian yellow curry noodle soup...................... 130

89. Malaysian Laksa noodle soup........................... 131

90. Instant Vietnamese pho..................................... 132

91. Thai Tom Yum vege soup.................................. 133

92. Thai Tom Yum noodle braise............................ 134

93. Hoisin, broccoli, noodle braise......................... 135

TINNED PINK SALMON.. 136

94. Pink salmon, creamy avo, chilli....................... 138

95. Pink salmon, spicy southern dressing.............139

96. Pink salmon, sauerkraut, gherkin.................... 140

97. Pink salmon, pineapple, capsicum................... 141

98. Pink salmon, mild chilli, lime.......................... 142

99. Pink salmon, dill, nori....................................... 143

100. Pink salmon, dill, Viet sauce........................144

101. Pink salmon, pickled ginger juice................ 145

102. Pink salmon, prawns, herbs, lime.................146

103. Pink salmon, prawns, pineapple, mint......... 147

104. Pink salmon, prawns, pineapple, ginger...... 148

105. Pink salmon, chilli, Viet mint...................... 149

106.	Pink salmon, coriander, Chang's	150
107.	Pink salmon, balsamic, coleslaw	151
108.	Pink salmon, tomato, mizuna	152
109.	Pink salmon, nori, mizuna	153
110.	Pink salmon, chilli, Thai basil	154
111.	Pink salmon, balsamic, coriander	155
112.	Pink salmon, nori, alfalfa, avo	156
113.	Pink salmon, coriander, lettuce	157
114.	Pink salmon, avo, jalapenos, lime	158
115.	Pink salmon, olives, basil, balsamic	159
116.	Pink salmon, Italian perfecto	160
117.	Pink salmon, guacamole	162
118.	Pink and smoked salmon, Chang's	163
119.	Pink salmon, jalapenos, mizuna	164
120.	Layered PINK salmon stir-fry	165

TINNED RED SALMON 167

121.	Red salmon, kaleslaw, jalapenos	168
122.	Red salmon, crunchy salad, ginger	169
123.	Red salmon, jalapenos, sesame oil	170
124.	Red salmon, Italian bruschetta	171
125.	Red salmon, ginger, kaleslaw	172
126.	Red salmon, cos lettuce, alfalfa	173
127.	Red salmon, avo, alfalfa, Caesar	174
128.	Red salmon, hot chilli, shallots	175

| 129. | Red salmon, avo, vinegar, herbs | 176 |
| 130. | Spicy red salmon salad bowl | 177 |

About the author...178

Titles in the HUNGER HERO DIET series......................179

Introduction

This recipe series showcases low-calorie and highly nutritious ways to prepare simple foods, following the principles of the ground-breaking HUNGER HERO DIET©.

Each of these special editions can be used as a standalone set of recipes, or as a companion to the original 300-page book:

The HUNGER HERO DIET©: How to Lose Weight and Break the Depression Cycle – Without Exercise, Drugs, or Surgery.

FISH is highly nutritious and low in calories – a perfect combination if you want to lose weight, lower blood pressure, lower triglycerides, reduce inflammation, increase HDL cholesterol, or improve insulin/glucose regulation. And the omega-3s help control appetite too (by improving *leptin* sensitivity) (Abete *et al.*, 2010). But too few people know how to prepare it.

In this instalment, we focus is on how to use TINNED FISH which is available in major Australian supermarkets. We help you navigate the myriad of tinned tuna and salmon on those shelves, so you can be sure of making healthy choices.

Most recipes are Vietnamese-inspired, focussing on flavour and texture, making the most of what we have in our fridge, pantry and freezer. Rice paper rolls and rice noodle dishes are a major feature, with lots of green leafy vegetables and herbs.

I lived for 10 years in an inner-city suburb of Melbourne, bustling with Vietnamese cafes and food markets. I learnt to appreciate the fresh and flavourful foods of SE Asia, using local produce, and once you get the hang of it, you'll be hooked too.

Each recipe is an original, created by me as I developed the HUNGER HERO DIET© and lost over 35kg in 35 weeks – without exercise, drugs, or surgery. As I experimented, I painstakingly recorded and photographed every meal. Rest assured that every image in this book is REAL and not photoshopped in any way. What you see is what you get.

The latest scientific evidence was used to select foods that are recognised for their health benefits, but they had to earn their place in the diet by providing the MOUTH with what it craves – foods with texture and flavour – crunchy, creamy, spicy, savory, salty, and umami.

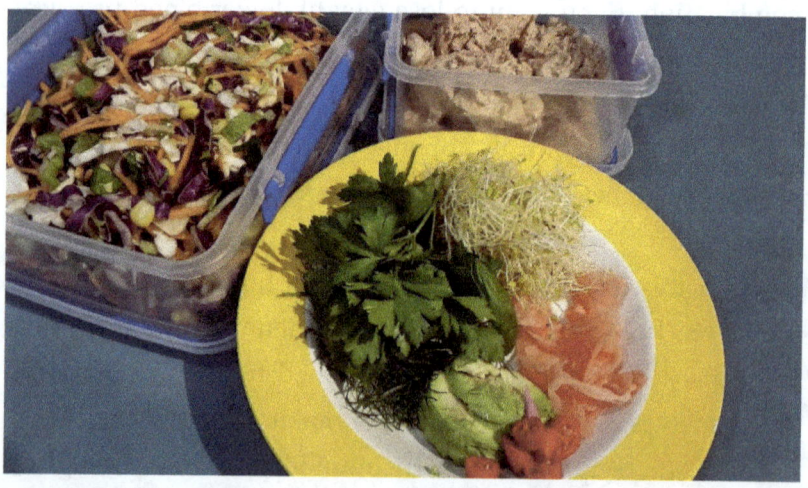

Foods were included, or omitted, for many reasons, but the end result was a beneficial mix of prebiotics, probiotics, macronutrients (protein, carbs, fats) and micronutrients (vitamins and minerals).

Many foods are repeated over and over, but the reason goes far beyond practicality and monetary economy. With a few simple tweaks, you can create multiple dishes with the same core ingredients. If you scroll down the following lists, you will see these foods appearing time and again. Most are 'functional foods' and packed full of nutrients.

Foods containing **WATER-SOLUBLE** vitamins:
- B1 (thiamine): Yeast, pork, cereal grains, sunflower seeds, brown rice, whole-grain rye, asparagus, kale, cauliflower, potatoes, oranges, liver, eggs.
- B2 (riboflavin): Asparagus, bananas, persimmons, okra, silverbeet, cottage cheese, ricotta cheese, milk, yoghurt, steak, eggs, fish, oysters, green beans.
- B3 (niacin): TUNA, beef liver, heart, kidney, chicken, beef, milk, eggs, avocados, dates, tomatoes, leafy greens, broccoli, carrots, sweet potatoes, asparagus, nuts, wholegrains, legumes, mushrooms, yeast.
- B5 (pantothenic acid): Egg yolk, liver, kidney, yeast, meats, wholegrains, broccoli, avocados, royal jelly, roe.
- B6 (pyridoxine): Chickpeas, steak, navy beans, liver, TUNA, salmon, chicken breast, bananas, cottage cheese.
- B7 (biotin): Egg yolk, liver, salmon, spinach, broccoli, yoghurt.
- B9 (folic acid): Leafy green vegetables, legumes (beans, lentils), asparagus, spinach, broccoli, avocado, mangoes, lettuce, sweet corn, liver, baker's yeast, sunflower seeds, citrus fruit.
- B12 (cyanocobalamin): Fish, shellfish, meat, poultry, eggs, dairy, and some fortified soy products.
- C (ascorbic acid): Guavas, capsicum, kiwifruit, strawberries, oranges, papayas, broccoli, tomatoes, kale, eggplant, snow peas.

Foods containing **FAT-SOLUBLE** vitamins:
- A (retinol, carotenoids): Liver, cod liver oil, carrots, broccoli, sweet potato, butter, kale, kiwi fruit, spinach, pumpkin, some cheeses, egg, apricot, cantaloupe melon, and milk. Our bodies convert the beta-carotene into vitamin A.
- D (ergocalciferol): There are traces in salmon, TUNA, sardines, oysters, prawns, egg yolks, mushrooms.
- E (tocopherols): Almonds, avocado, eggs, milk, nuts, leafy greens, unheated vegetable oils, wheat germ, wholegrains.
- K (phylloquinone): Leafy greens such as kale, silverbeet, Asian greens, parsley. Vitamin K helps vitamin E with normal blood clotting and wound healing.

How to make rice paper rolls

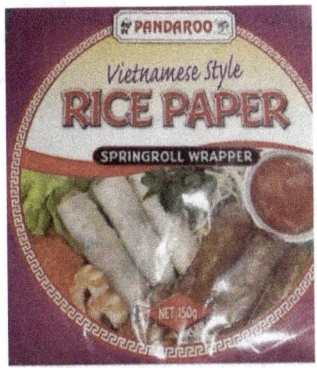

Pandaroo Vietnamese Style Rice Paper, spring roll wrappers, 10 large round sheets per pack

For the weight conscious, these rice paper rounds help maintain correct portion size, and the unique combination of tapioca and rice flours can reduce appetite. When the dry papers are reconstituted in a water bath, the soft pliable wrappers take on a gelatinous feel, and when you eat them, your gut registers a pleasant sense of fullness.

To make our rice paper rolls, you will need a pack of dried rice paper rounds, a serve of protein, creamy Greek yoghurt, sweet and spicy sushi ginger, a touch of chili heat, a cup of mixed coleslaw vegetables (such as cabbage, carrot, celery, onion), a few baby lettuce leaves, some aromatic Asian herbs, and a few slices of avocado when they're in season and not costing a fortune!

Our Vietnamese-inspired gluten-free rice paper rolls are a perfect combination of flavours and textures – smooth, chewy, creamy, sour, spicy, crunchy, sweet and aromatic. They contain all the food groups, with the added benefit of being *prebiotic* (coleslaw) and *probiotic* (natural Greek yoghurt).

METHOD
1. Get organised. Place all ingredients and utensils on a clean kitchen bench. If you can, sit down at the bench too, as this makes it easier to roll the rice papers.
2. Set aside THREE sheets of rice paper (dinner plate size)
3. Place a large flat plate or tray on the bench. Must be large enough to allow for a sheet of rice paper to be submerged in water.
4. Add a little room-temperature tap water to the large plate. (Do not use warm water or the rice paper will soften too quickly.)
5. Submerge one sheet of rice paper in the water. Give it a little poke with your finger to keep it under water for a few seconds. Before it goes limp, lift it out, and lay it flat on a plastic cutting board, or kitchen bench.
6. Quickly build the filling on one side of the wet wrapper, before it becomes too limp to manage. Add wet ingredients first, and finish with dry salad – it acts as a protective cover and makes it less messy to roll up.
7. When you have a little mound of filling neatly arranged on the rice paper, carefully lift the nearest edge and fold over to cover the filling. By starting at the front, you can then fold the sides, and finish by rolling it to the other end. You should have a neat parcel. Repeat.

HINT: Wet rice paper quickly softens to become limp and sticky, so don't be surprised if your first few attempts look untidy. If you make a mess, don't give up; just wrap the whole thing in a large lettuce leaf to hold it together. You will get better with practice, and patience. The trick is to wet one rice paper at a time, get the filling done quickly, and roll it up before the wrapper becomes too soft and sticky.

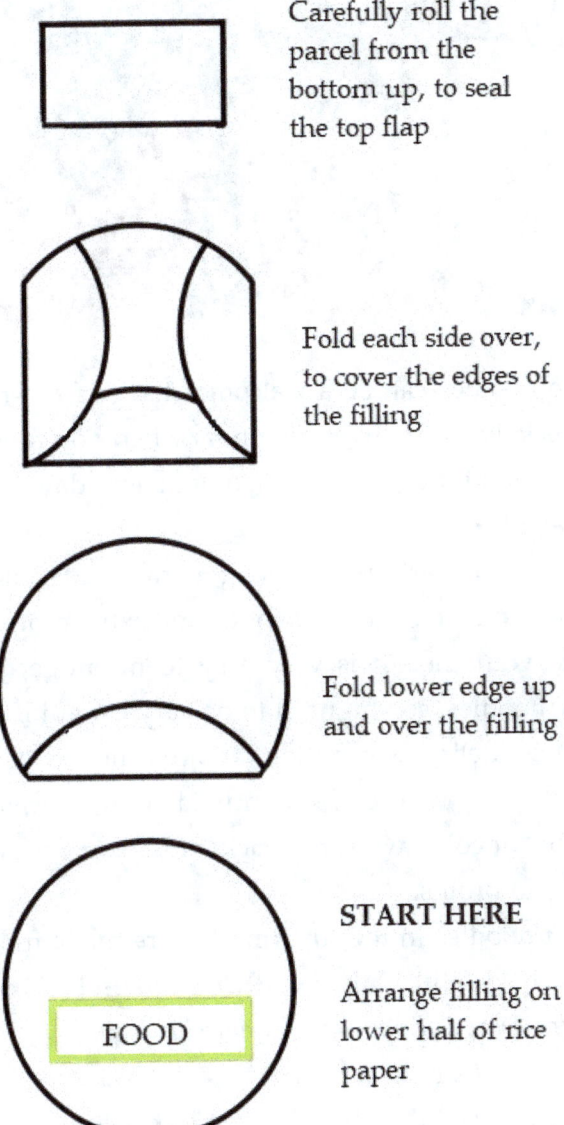

How to prepare rice noodles

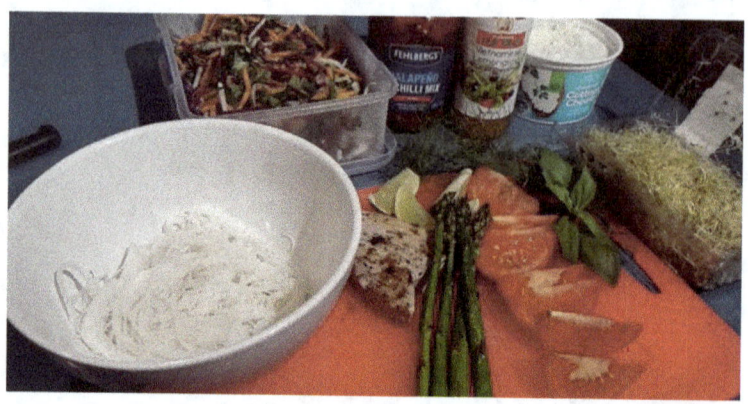

Rice noodles can be a welcome change from rice paper rolls, especially in the winter months when you're wanting a hot plate of food. But don't eat noodles every day if you want to lose weight.

Once you start freewheeling with salads and noodle bowls, you can become heavy handed and extra calories quickly creep into your diet. It is very easy to misjudge quantities, especially noodles, so you need to be very careful if you want to enjoy these delicious variations and continue to lose weight.

Most recipes use reconstituted thin vermicelli rice noodles (hot or cold), while the thicker ribbon noodles are ideal for soups and broths.

Most noodles in the supermarket are made from wheat, not rice, so be careful. Only buy RICE noodles. For example:.

- **Wai Wai Bihoon** Rice Vermicelli, plain, pack of 10x50g bundles, 182cals, and
- **Erawan** Pad Thai Rice Noodles (thick ribbons)

OPTIONAL *(These are higher in calories, so be careful):*
- **Wai Wai** Noodles, Rice Vermicelli Instant, with crab-flavoured sachets, in a packet, 55g, 211cals, or
- **Lian** Pho Ga Vietnamese Style instant rice noodles, 70g, with flavour sachets, in a plastic bowl

What does a single serve of noodles look like?

A 500g packet of **Wai Wai Bihoon Rice Vermicelli noodles** contains 10 bundles of dry noodles, each weighing 50g. That's about 180 calories – way too much carbohydrate if you're trying to lose weight or maintain your weight loss. To keep total calories for a meal within appropriate limits, the rice noodle component should not exceed 100 calories.

To achieve this, it's very simple. Take a pair of large kitchen scissors, snip each bundle in half, then store the dried noodles in a large plastic container in the pantry. You now have 20 little bundles of noodles, each one a proper serving size, ready to add to your meals.

Flat ribbon noodles are not so quick and easy. But with a little planning, it can be done. Read the label and calculate what a single serve would look like. As with the vermicelli noodles, the packaging on thicker 'rice sticks' or ribbon noodles also recommends 50g as the serving size. But at 180 calories, this is too much. Again, try to limit your serving size to 100 calories.

There are many different brands of thick ribbon rice noodles, but the pack in front of me right now weighs 375g, with 8 serves at 50g each. If we reduce serving size to 100 calories, that equates to about 28g per serve, or about 13 serves to a packet of noodles instead of only 8.

There is no way around it. In this instance, I need to weigh out 28g of ribbon noodles for a single serve. And because I despise having to weigh my food, I do all the weighing in one go, to get it over and done with while I'm in the mood to be finicky – which isn't often!

For efficiency and convenience, I weigh out 28g and pop them into a resealable sandwich bag. When I'm done, I'll have about 13 little packets, which I then place in a large plastic storage container (with the empty packet, so I know what they are) and store in the pantry until needed. Easy-peasy.

How to reconstitute thin vermicelli rice noodles

Thin rice noodles are quick and easy to prepare:
- Place a single serve (25g) of dry vermicelli noodles into a bowl, cover with boiling water, then give a little stir
- Place a lid or plate over the bowl to keep the heat in
- After a few minutes, take a look, and give them a little stir. They should be plump and soft. Drain. Depending on the recipe, the noodles can be served warm with a cooked dish or chilled in the fridge and added to a salad.

HINT: If planning to make a soup, don't drain the noodles. Stir a teaspoon of stock powder (or miso) into the hot water, add some chopped leafy Asian greens, and a few thin slices of a favourite protein. Cover the bowl again for a few minutes to allow the extras to cook, but you can zap in the microwave for a couple of minutes if you want it piping hot. Season to taste.

How to reconstitute flat ribbon rice noodles

These noodles are thicker than vermicelli, so they need to be cooked in boiling water on the stove for a few minutes.

- Pour a few cups of water into a saucepan, place on the stove, and bring to the boil
- Add a single serve (25-28g) of dried flat noodles (make sure there's enough hot water to submerge the noodles). Leave the pan uncovered.
- After a few minutes, take a look, and give them a little stir. They should be plump and soft. Remove from stove and drain.

HINT: If making soup, leave saucepan on stove and don't drain noodles. Stir in a teaspoon of stock powder (or miso), add a handful of chopped leafy greens, and a few thin slices of a favourite protein. Cover and simmer for a couple of minutes. Remove from heat. Pour everything into a soup bowl. Season to taste.

How to eat the rainbow

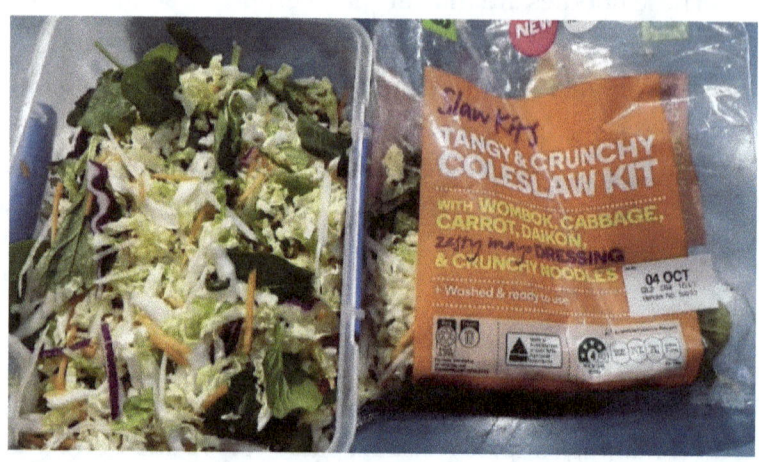

The public health message being yelled from rooftops for decades has been, "EAT THE RAINBOW". But most of us either ignore it, or don't fully understand how to do it.

For most of us, vegetables are a chore. We might have a few favourites that we eat regularly, but how many of us eat RED, YELLOW, ORANGE, WHITE, and GREEN on a daily basis? Not many, I'll wager, and not without help.

And if we do think to buy a variety of vegetables, they sit in the bottom crisper until they shrivel into nothingness, because we don't know what to do with them, and really couldn't be bothered. Not only is that wasting precious food, but wasting money too.

As a single person with only myself to feed, this scenario was all too common. Then I stumbled across all the pre-cut and pre-packaged SALADS covering numerous shelves in the chilled section of my local supermarket.

They have come a long way from the days when the only choice was a bag of Greek or Caesar Salad. These old favourites still exist, but there are so many more choices these days – and they are changing all the time.

Every major supermarket chain in Australia has their own selection of pre-packaged salads and slaw kits, but these were from my local store. I was very happy with their extensive selection, but all supermarkets change and update their products over time, with seasonal availability of produce, and in line with consumer trends. Here are some of the packs I experimented with while developing recipes for the HUNGER HERO DIET:

- Woolworth's Crunchy Noodle Coleslaw Kit
- Woolworth's Slaw Kits, Creamy Classic Coleslaw Kit,
- Woolworth's Classic Coleslaw
- Woolworth's Fine Cut Coleslaw
- Woolworth's Four Seasons Coleslaw
- Woolworth's Slaw Kits Kaleslaw
- Woolworth's Asian Style Salad Kit
- Woolworth's Thai Salad Kit (red cabbage, carrot, capsicum, celery, mizuna lettuce, with packs of Thai style dressing and crispy fried onion flakes)

Once I discovered all these salad kits, I soon realised how even a subtle change of vegetables or dressings could completely alter the flavour profile of a salad. Without realising it, I was EATING THE RAINBOW, and loving it.

These packs have all sorts of names, but the ones that provide a core element in all the recipes in this series, and in THE HUNGER HERO DIET©, are generally a slaw – featuring some type of shredded cabbage (European green, red, or Asian wombok), with shredded carrot, sliced onion, chopped shallots, and celery. Others include interesting variations such as grated raw beetroot, corn kernels, or Mizuna lettuce.

I suggest starting with a basic coleslaw mix, such as the Crunchy Noodle Coleslaw kit, then try a few other packs to add variety. You can also mix them together to create something new. As you will see from the recipes in this book, I often combined kaleslaw with other coleslaw packs to include a wider range of vegetables in every meal.

I had thought these packs were an expensive indulgence, but then I realised how far one pack could stretch. After a few days of adding fresh salad vegetables to meals, I added the remaining bits to whatever I was cooking, even the lettuce and other salad greens! Now I do this all the time, and good food was never so easy.

NB: Most salad packs contain extra sachets of salad dressings and crunchy toppings. These are extra calories you don't need. Keep a couple in the kitchen door for occasional use, or when a recipe suggests you use them, but bin the rest.

How to add flavour

The rough translation for **kuchisabishii** is 'lonely mouth', and this Japanese expression describes why we MINDLESSLY feed our mouths – by smoking, eating, or drinking. A 'lonely mouth' can cause havoc, so we need to keep it happy, without stuffing things into it all the time.

The recipes in the original HUNGER HERO DIET©, and in this companion series, focus on keeping our mouth happy.

It sounds counter-intuitive, but we need to give our mouth what it wants – or at least something that satisfies the specific craving. Those desires might be **textural** (crunchy, crispy, smooth, creamy, liquid, chewy, soft, sticky) or **flavourful** (sweet, sour, bitter, salty, spicy, savoury/umami).

The major food groups provide most of the textural elements – the seafood proteins, the rice paper wrappers, rice noodles, and the vegetables. But most of the flavours will come from things we add, such as cooking sauces and condiments. Here are a few of my favourites, many of which feature in these recipes. You can gain inspiration from what you keep in your fridge door or pantry.

COOKING SAUCES

- Australian or Italian extra virgin olive oil, cold pressed
- **Valcom** Authentic Thai Tom Yum paste (gives a fragrant, spicy chili hit)
- **Valcom** Authentic Thai Pad Thai stir-fry paste (very mild and a little sweet)

- **Jeeny's Oriental Foods** Tamarind Puree, 220g (adds a sour umami-like element to counteract sweetness and adds depth to spicy dishes)
- **Vegeta** vegetable-flavoured powdered stock
- **Hikari** Japanese Miso Instant Soup with Wakame seaweed, 12 sachets to a pack (a quick way to add depth of flavour to soups)
- Hoisin, oyster, and plum sauces
- Passata or pasta sauce
- Light soy sauce and fish sauce can be used to enhance cooking or as a table condiment

CONDIMENTS

- Iodised salt
- Freshly cracked pepper
- A jar of Pickled jalapenos, sliced
- **Conimex** Sambal Oelek hot chilli paste
- **Trident** Hot Chilli Sauce
- **Pandaroo** Sushi Ginger, 200g jar

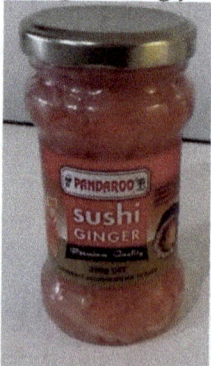

- **Poonsin** Vietnamese Spring Roll Dipping Sauce, 300ml (perfect for all seafood dishes and salads)
- **Chang's** Crispy Noodle Salad Dressing, 280ml (you can taste the hint of sesame oil and soy sauce)
- **ABC** Kecap Manis sweet soy sauce
- Japanese **Obentu** brand Tonkatsu Sauce

FRESH HERBS

Fresh herbs play an important role in Asian cuisine. Many are seasonal, so not always available in supermarkets. But they are easy to grow at home in pots on a balcony.

- Coriander
- Dill
- Fennel
- Parsley
- Thai basil
- Vietnamese mint

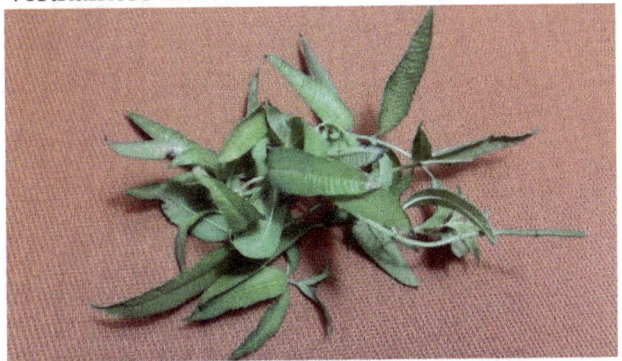

BASIC RICE PAPER ROLLS

The standard rice paper roll recipe across the HUNGER HERO DIET SERIES consists of:

- moistened rice paper,
- a protein, usually seafood, but pork or tofu sometimes,
- Greek yoghurt as a fermented probiotic food, but also providing a creamy element,
- ¼ avocado for creamy texture and unsaturated fats,
- chilli or jalapenos for hot spicy,
- pickled pink sushi ginger for sweet spicy,
- fresh herbs for extra flavour and micro-nutrients,
- mixed salad for micro-nutrients and crunch.

You will be amazed at how different each recipe becomes by changing only one or two ingredients each time. Once you get the hang of it, you can mix and match all sorts of foods. You are only limited by your imagination. But if your aim is to lose weight, don't stray too far off the path.

Don't use any dressing on the salads unless the recipe says to do so. The Greek yoghurt provides the creamy element without anything artificial, and the occasional slice of avocado adds an extra smooth richness. Try to keep every dish clean and fresh, with a combination of flavours and textures. Keep your mouth happy.

TINNED TUNA

Yellowfin TUNA is an excellent source of protein, omega-3s, phosphorous, vitamins B3, B12 and D, and a rich source of selenium – which helps reduce inflammation and oxidative stress (free radicals).

Tuna has become so popular that supermarkets carry multiple brands and dozens of variations, but the main players are:

- Tuna in springwater
- Tuna in brine
- Tuna in oil, or
- Minced tuna with added flavourings.

Avoid the tiny 95g tins of flavoured tuna, such as sweet chilli, spicy chilli, mayonnaise and corn, chilli and beans, laksa, Indian curry, etc. The tuna is mushy, it won't satisfy your appetite, and it adds extra calories. However, it doesn't hurt to keep a couple at the back of the kitchen cupboard for the occasional treat when you go hunting for something different. Spread on a couple of rice cakes for a mid-afternoon snack, but not too often, as these flavoured tins are high in calories and tend to increase your appetite instead of managing it.

TUNA in SPRINGWATER is your staple lunch protein if you are looking to reduce calories and lose weight. But there are many different brands to choose from – with variations in texture, smell, taste, and price.

I've tried many different brands, but my personal favourite is **WOOLWORTH'S** Yellowfin Tuna in Springwater. It has good colour, firm texture, a mild flavour, and is one of the cheapest. It comes in 425g, 185g, and 95g tins.

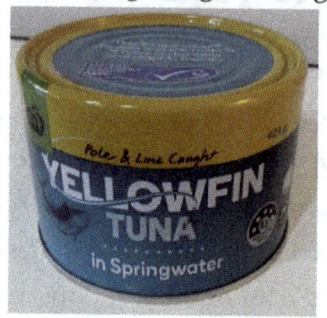

I prefer the larger 425g tins because they contain larger chunks, and leftovers will keep in a plastic container for a few days in the fridge. Consider the Goldilocks Effect – 95g is too small for a single serve, and 185g is too much, but the 425g is just right (enough for 3 meals).

NB: Supply chain issues post-covid have struck hard, and the larger tins have been unavailable recently. I don't know if they will return to shelves, so you might need to go with the smaller tins or undertake your own research and try a few brands until you find your personal favourite.

TUNA ROLLS with all the basics

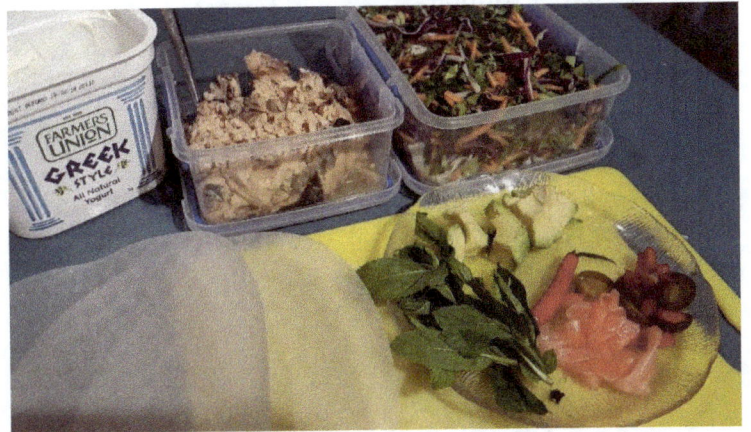

1. Tuna, ginger, avo, Asian slaw

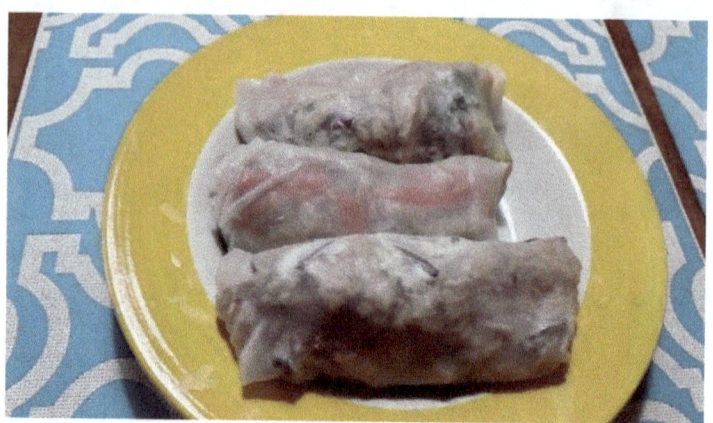

- 3 rice paper rounds
- 150g tinned tuna in springwater, drained
- A few teaspoons of Greek yoghurt
- ¼ avocado
- A few strips of Pandaroo Sushi Ginger
- Pickled jalapenos, sliced
- Cup of Asian Coleslaw kit, dry (no dressing)

2. Tuna, sambal, kaleslaw

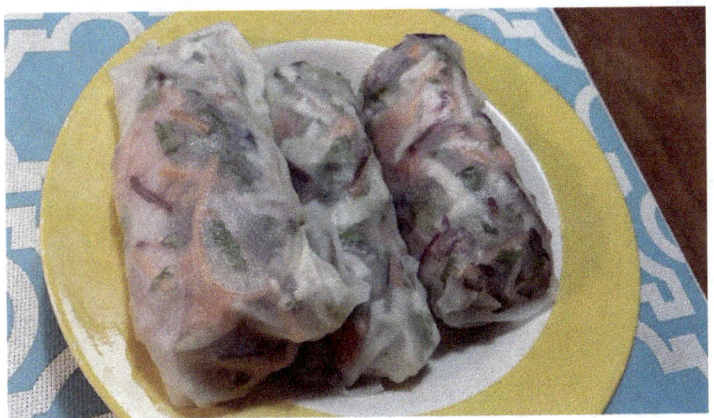

- 3 rice paper rounds
- 150g tinned tuna in springwater, drained
- Greek yoghurt
- ¼ avocado
- Conimex Sambal Oelek chili paste
- Pandaroo Sushi Ginger
- Kaleslaw

3. Tuna, avo, mixed slaw

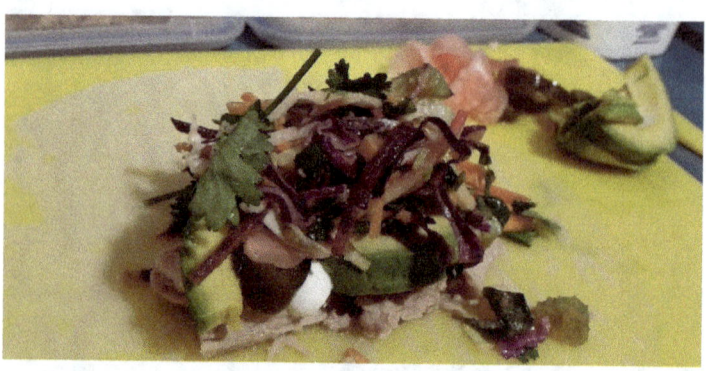

- 3 rice paper rounds
- 150g tinned tuna in springwater, drained
- Greek yoghurt
- ¼ avocado
- Pandaroo Sushi Ginger
- Pickled jalapenos, sliced
- Mixed coleslaw/kaleslaw (dry)

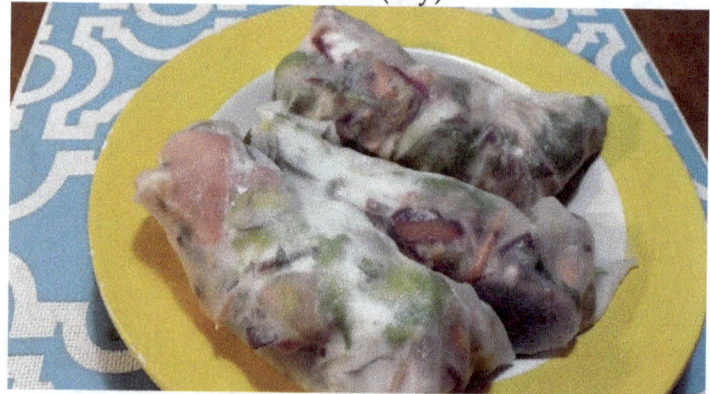

4. Tuna, chilli, avo, kaleslaw

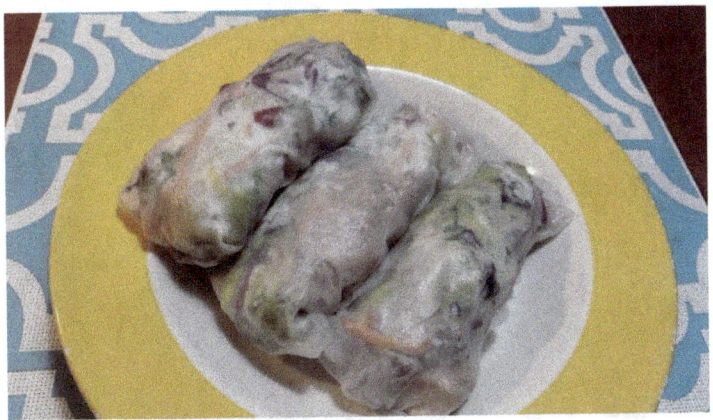

- 3 rice paper rounds
- 150g tinned tuna in springwater, drained
- Greek yoghurt
- ¼ avocado
- Chopped red chilli
- Chopped green chilli
- Kaleslaw (dry)

5. Tuna, spicy slaw, onion flakes

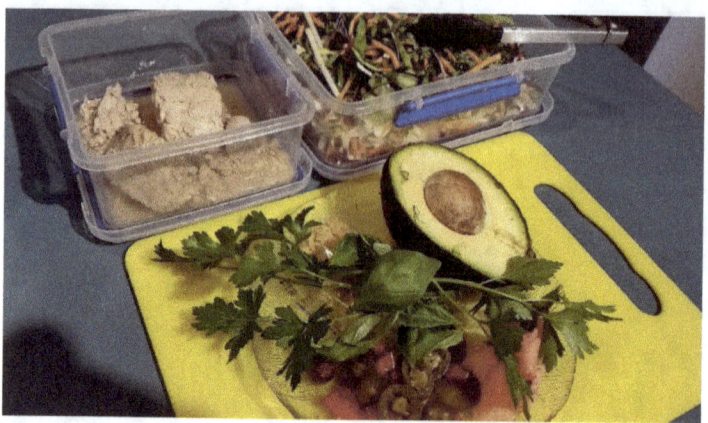

- 3 rice paper rounds
- 150g tinned tuna in springwater, drained
- Greek yoghurt
- ¼ avocado
- Pandaroo Sushi Ginger
- Pickled jalapenos, sliced
- Chilli
- Southern Style coleslaw/kaleslaw (dry)
- Fresh herbs (basil, parsley)
- Sprinkle fried onion flakes

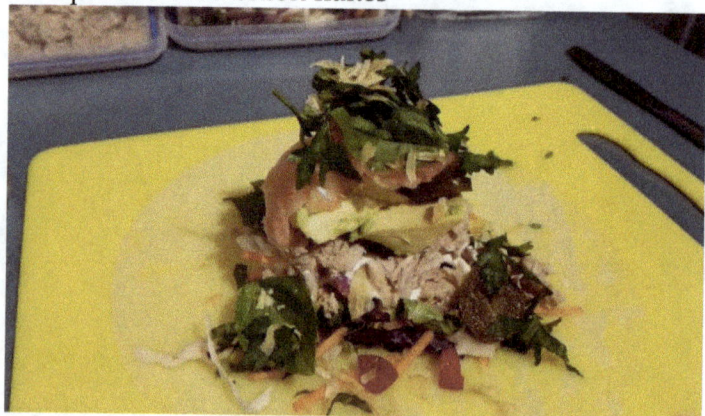

6. Tuna, chilli, dill, kaleslaw

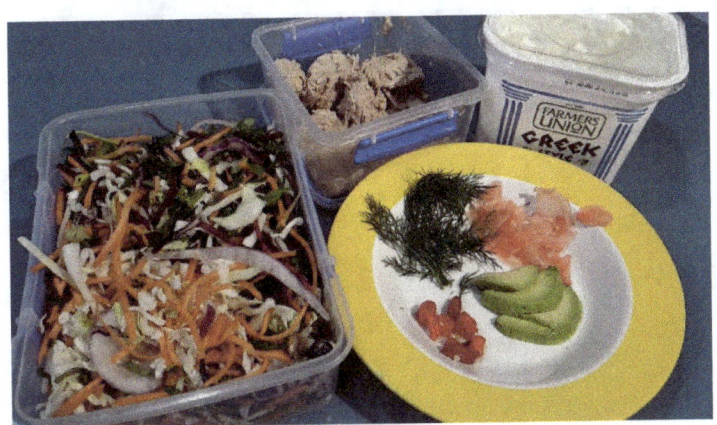

- 3 rice paper rounds
- 150g tinned tuna in springwater, drained
- Greek yoghurt
- ¼ avocado
- Pandaroo Sushi Ginger
- Chopped red chilli
- Mixed coleslaw/kaleslaw (dry)
- Fresh dill

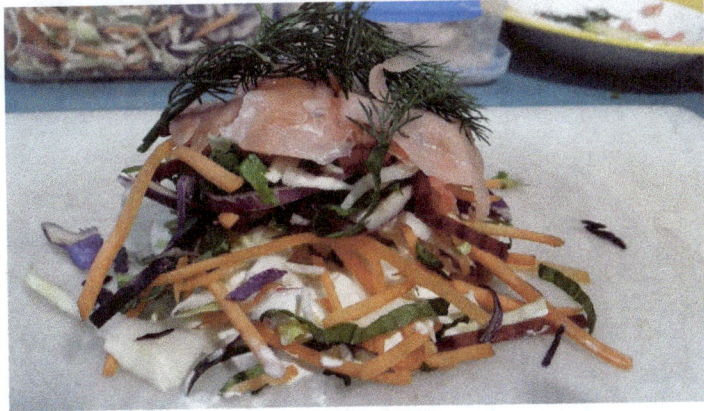

7. Tuna, sambal, Thai mizuna

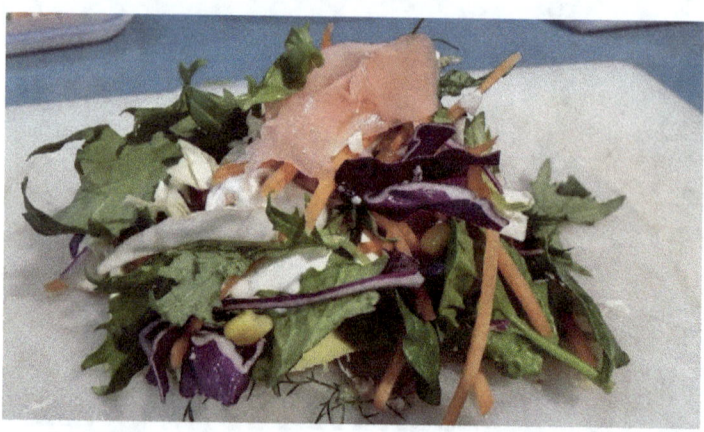

- 3 rice paper rounds
- 150g tinned tuna in springwater, drained
- Greek yoghurt
- ¼ avocado
- Pandaroo Sushi Ginger
- Teaspoon of Conimex Sambal Oelek
- Lemon juice
- Mixed coleslaw/Thai mizuna salad kit (dry)
- Fresh herbs (Thai basil, Viet mint, parsley, fennel)

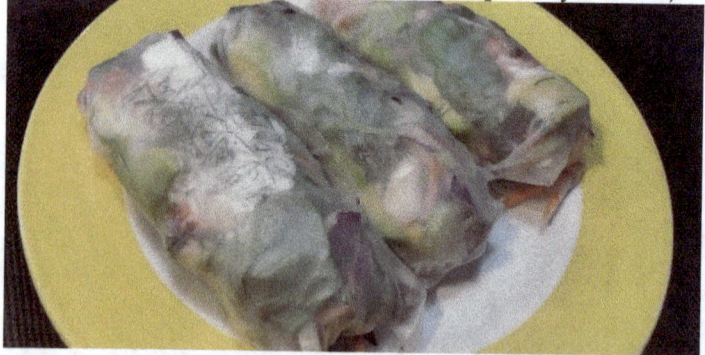

8. Tuna, Trident chilli, herbs

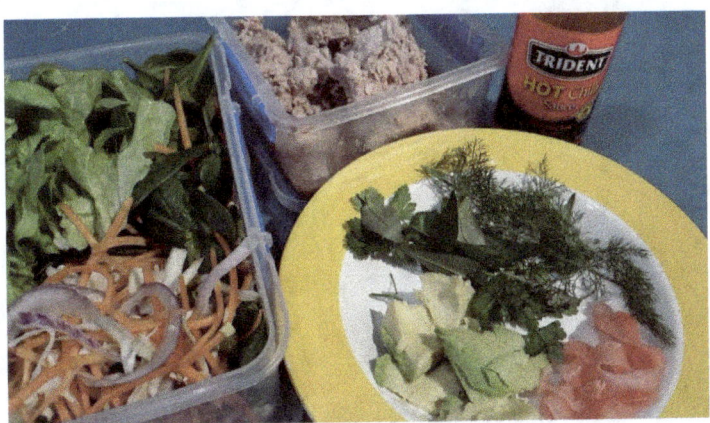

- 3 rice paper rounds
- 150g tinned tuna in springwater, drained
- Greek yoghurt
- ¼ avocado
- Pandaroo Sushi Ginger
- Trident Hot Chilli Sauce
- Crunchy Coleslaw Salad with onion rings (dry)
- Baby leaf salad
- Fresh herbs (Viet mint, parsley, fennel)

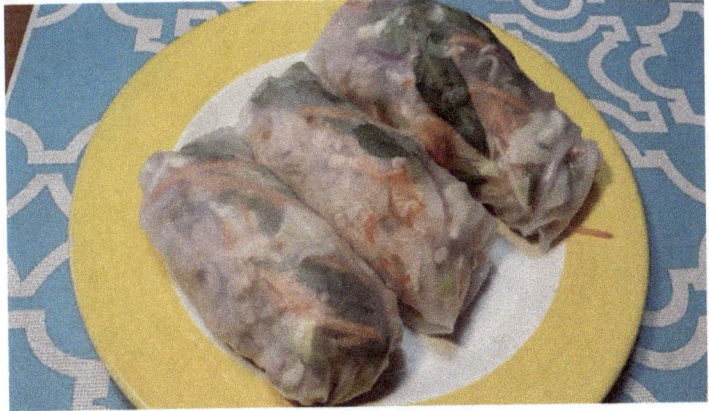

9. Tuna, Asian salad slaw

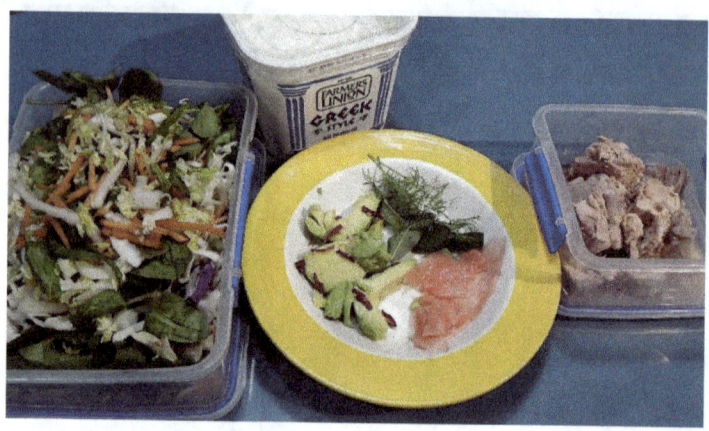

- 3 rice paper rounds
- 150g tinned tuna in springwater, drained
- Greek yoghurt
- ¼ avocado
- Pandaroo Sushi Ginger
- Teaspoon fresh chopped red chili
- Mixed baby leaves
- Asian vegetable slaw, dry
- Fresh herbs (Vietnamese mint, fennel)

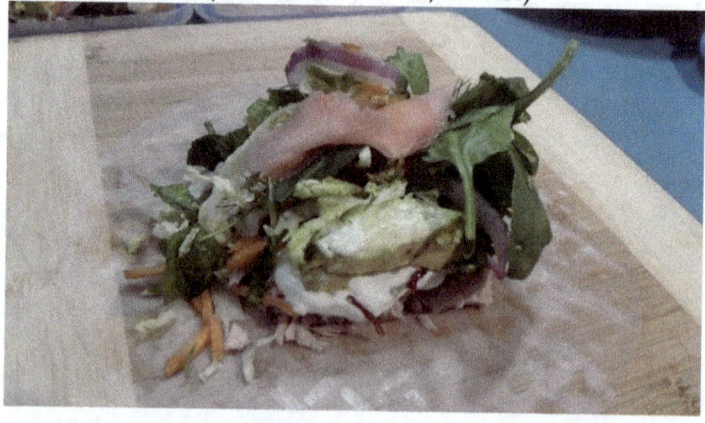

10. Tuna, Sambal, Oakleaf

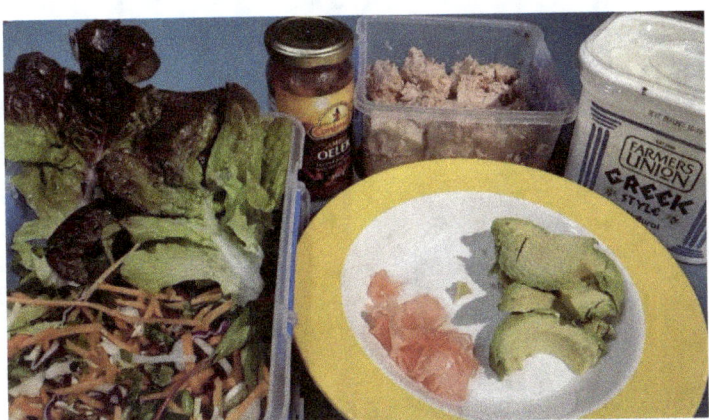

- 3 rice paper rounds
- 150g tinned tuna in springwater, drained
- Greek yoghurt
- ¼ avocado
- Pandaroo Sushi Ginger
- Teaspoon of Conimex Sambal Oelek
- Kaleslaw (dry)
- Oakleaf lettuce

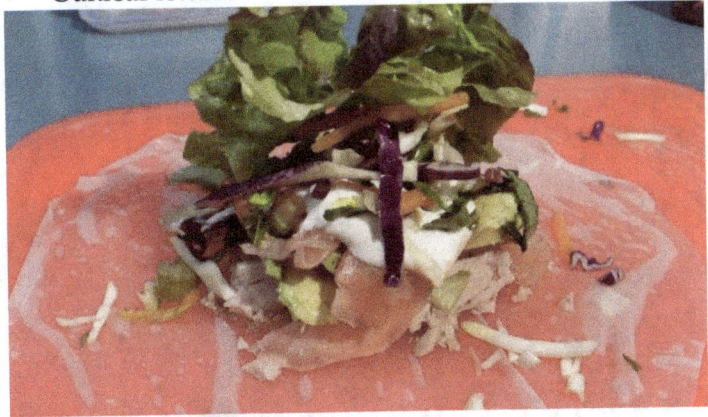

11. Tuna, Gochujang, lemon thyme

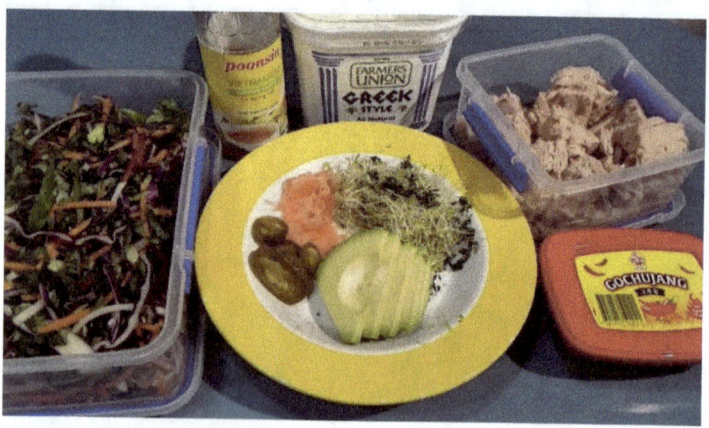

- 3 rice paper rounds
- 150g tinned tuna in springwater, drained
- Greek yoghurt
- ¼ avocado
- Pandaroo Sushi Ginger
- Pickled jalapenos, sliced
- Gochujang chilli paste (very mild chilli)
- Alfalfa sprouts
- Mixed kaleslaw/Thai Mizuna Salad kit
- Fresh lemon thyme
- Poonsin Vietnamese Spring Roll Dipping Sauce

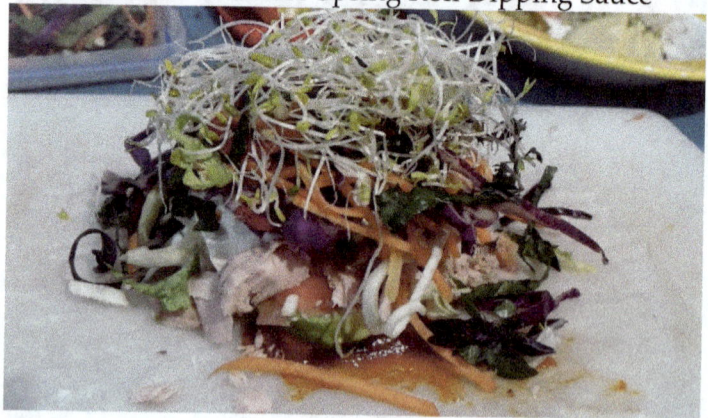

12. Tuna, sambal, mint, fennel

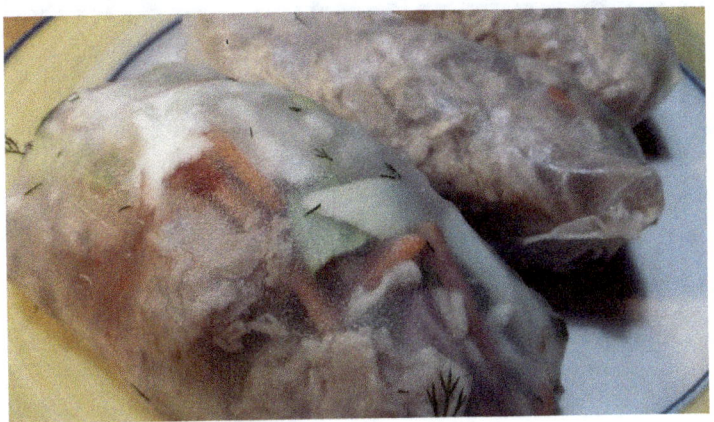

- 3 rice paper rounds
- 150g tinned tuna in springwater, drained
- Greek yoghurt
- ¼ avocado
- Pandaroo Sushi Ginger
- Conimex Sambal Oelek
- Mixed coleslaw/kaleslaw
- Alfalfa sprouts
- Fresh herbs (Vietnamese mint, parsley, fennel)

13. Tuna, sambal, coleslaw, lime

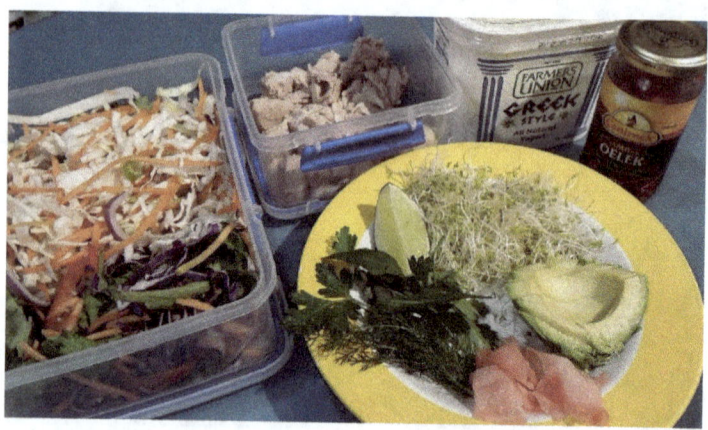

- 3 rice paper rounds
- 150g tinned tuna in springwater, drained
- Greek yoghurt
- ¼ avocado
- Pandaroo Sushi Ginger
- Lime juice
- Conimex Sambal Oelek
- Mixed Crunchy Coleslaw/kaleslaw
- Fresh herbs (Vietnamese mint, parsley, fennel)

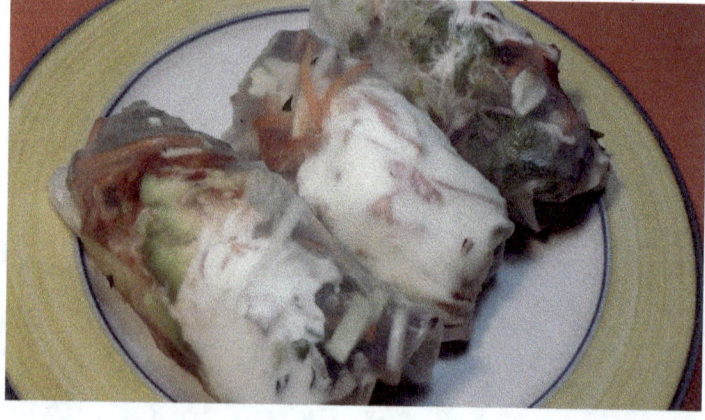

14. Tuna, avo, beetroot, fennel

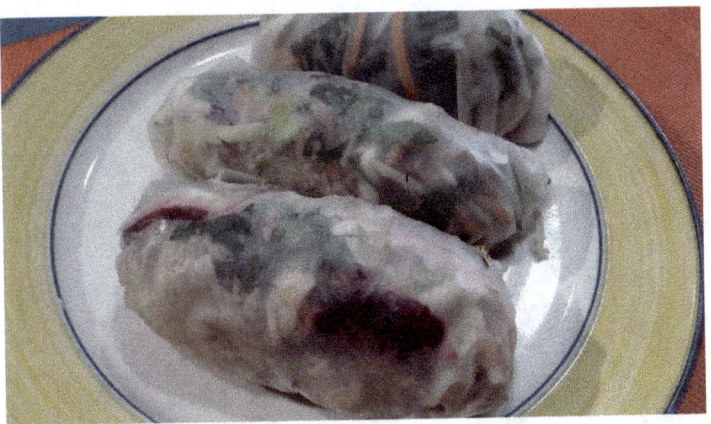

- 3 rice paper rounds
- 150g tinned tuna in springwater, drained
- Greek yoghurt
- ¼ avocado
- Pandaroo Sushi Ginger
- Pickled beetroot, sliced
- Teaspoon fresh chopped green chili (hot)
- Mixed lettuce
- Crunchy Coleslaw salad kit, dry
- Fresh herbs (parsley, fennel)

15. Tuna, guacamole, kaleslaw

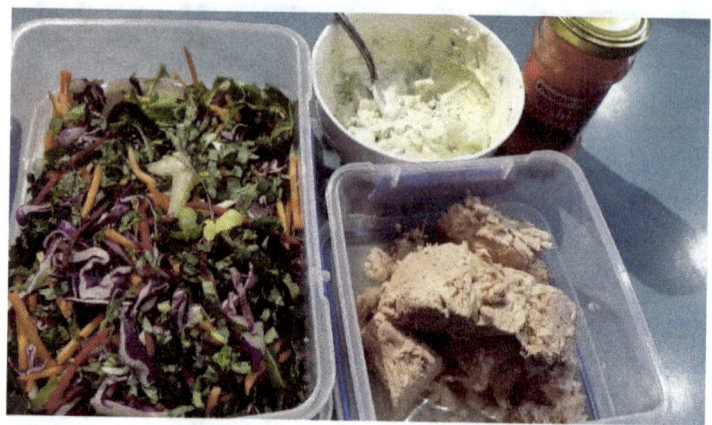

- 3 rice paper rounds
- 150g tinned tuna in springwater, drained
- To make guacamole – mix together,
    - Greek yoghurt
    - ¼ avocado
    - Conimex Sambal Oelek chilli
    - ½ onion, chopped
    - Fresh parsley
- Pandaroo Sushi Ginger
- Lime juice
- Kaleslaw

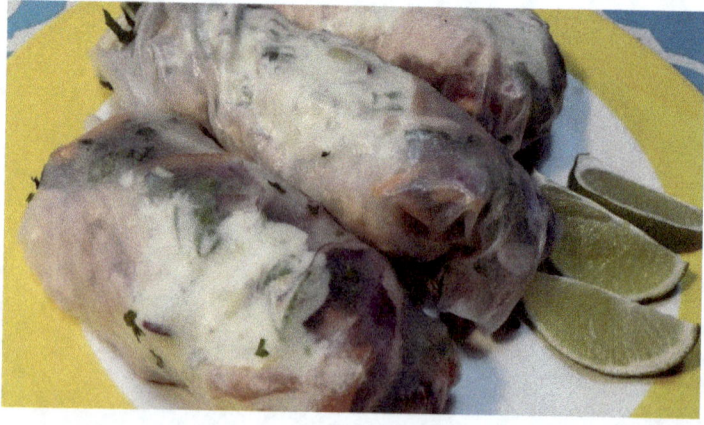

16. Tuna, kaleslaw, alfalfa

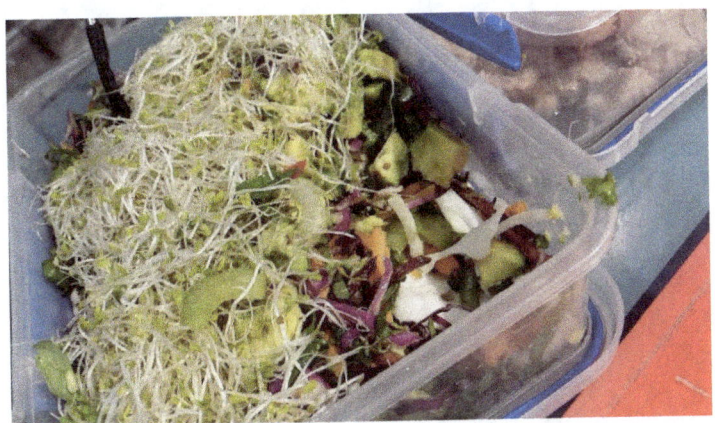

- 3 rice paper rounds
- 150g tinned tuna in springwater, drained
- Greek yoghurt
- ¼ avocado
- Pandaroo Sushi Ginger
- Lemon juice
- Mixed kale/coleslaw
- Baby lettuce leaves
- Alfalfa sprouts

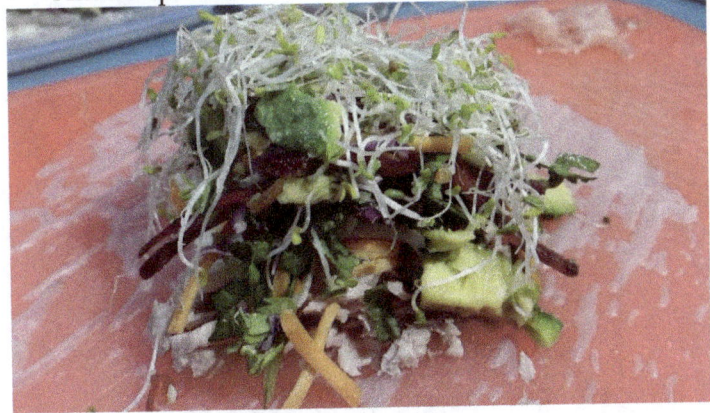

17. Tuna, vinegar, jalapenos, Viet mint

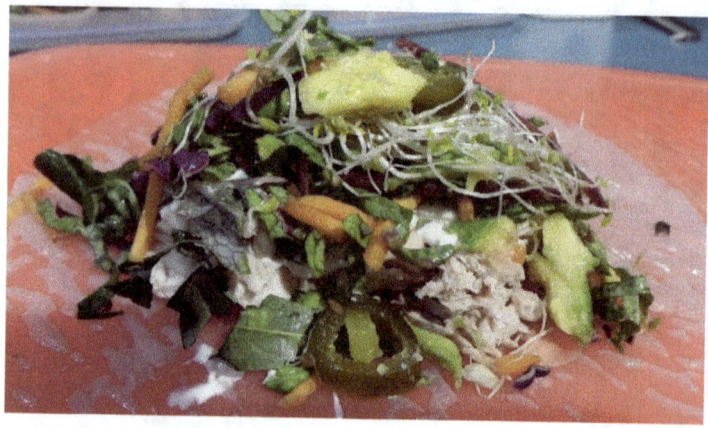

- 3 rice paper rounds
- 150g tinned tuna in springwater, drained
- Greek yoghurt
- ¼ avocado
- Pandaroo Sushi Ginger
- Splash of apple cider vinegar
- Pickled jalapenos, chopped
- Red chilli, chopped
- Mixed kale/coleslaw
- Alfalfa sprouts
- Fresh Vietnamese mint

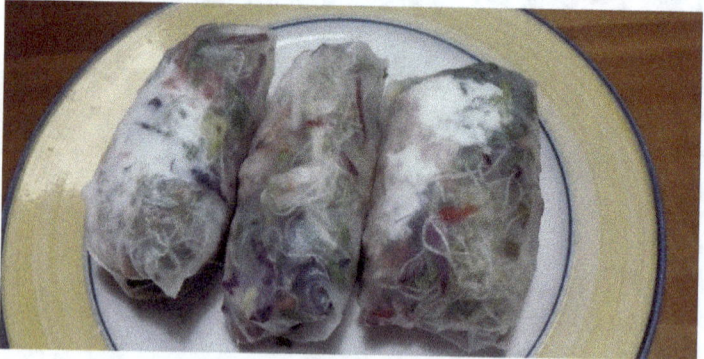

18. Tuna, dill, dried onion flakes

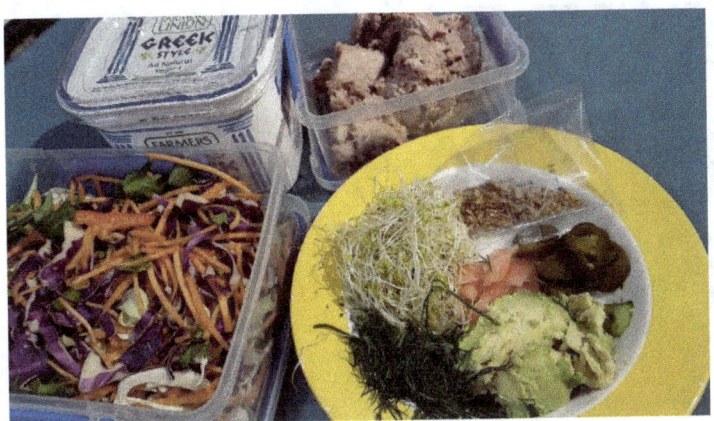

- 3 rice paper rounds
- 150g tinned tuna in springwater, drained
- Greek yoghurt
- ¼ avocado
- Pandaroo Sushi Ginger
- Pickled jalapenos, sliced
- Mixed Crunchy Coleslaw/Thai Mizuna Salad kit
- Fresh dill
- Alfalfa sprouts
- Crunchy dried onion flakes (from the salad kit)

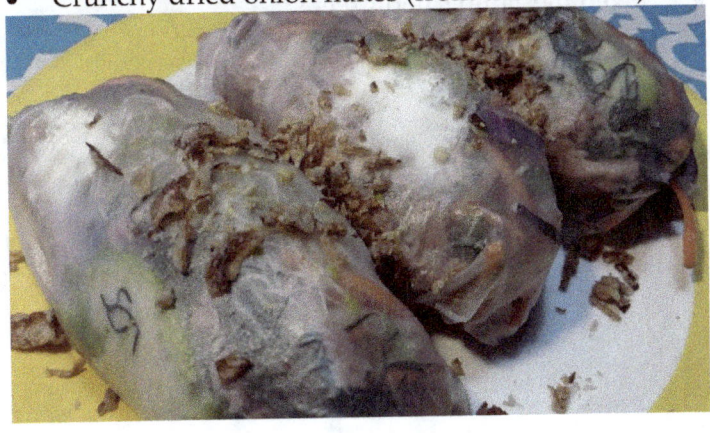

19. Tuna, Fukujinzuke, pea sprouts

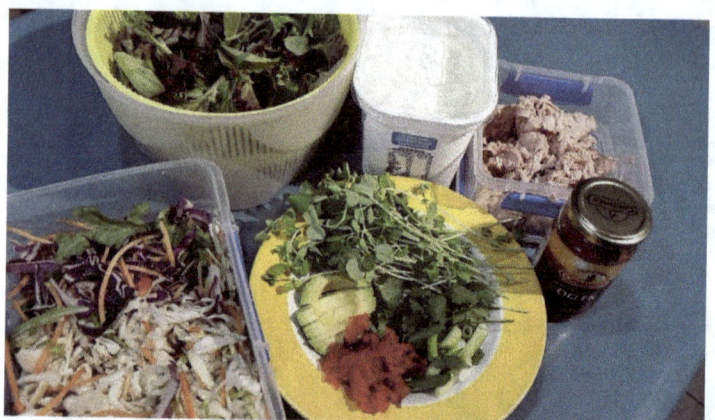

What's new? Snow pea sprouts instead of alfalfa, coriander instead of Vietnamese mint, with fresh shallots. Pea sprouts made it taste very GREEN, maybe too much. Work in progress.

- 3 rice paper rounds
- 150g tinned tuna in springwater, drained
- Greek yoghurt
- ¼ avocado
- Fukujinzuke (Japanese sweet pickled vegetables)
- Conimex Sambal Oelek
- Mixed mesculin salad greens
- Mixed Crunchy Coleslaw/Kaleslaw
- Chopped shallots
- Snow pea sprouts
- Fresh coriander

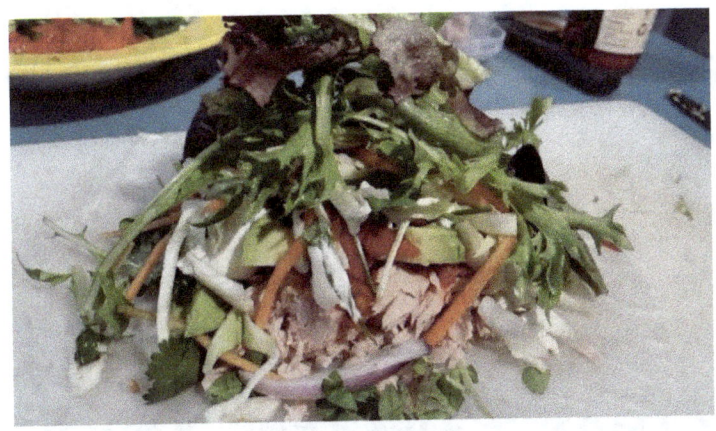

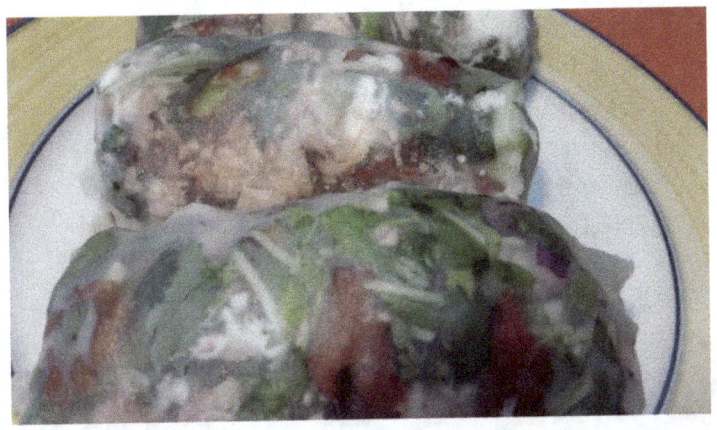

20. Tuna, Fukujinzuke, shallots, mint

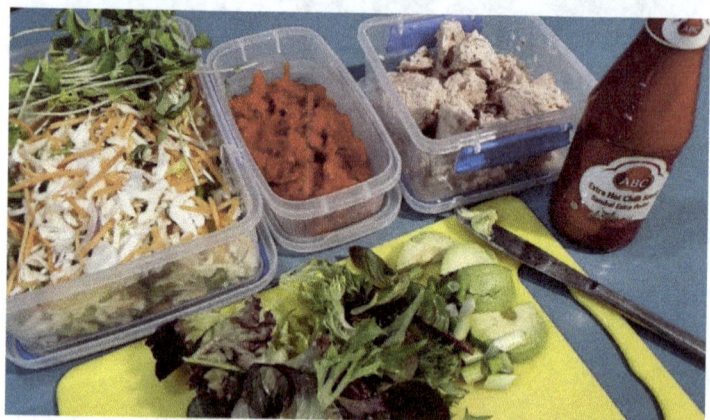

- 3 rice paper rounds
- 150g tinned tuna in springwater, drained
- Greek yoghurt
- ¼ avocado
- Fukujinzuke (Japanese sweet pickled vegetables)
- ABC very hot chilli sauce
- Mixed mesculin salad greens
- Crunchy Coleslaw veg, dry
- Chopped shallots
- Snow pea sprouts
- Fresh Vietnamese mint

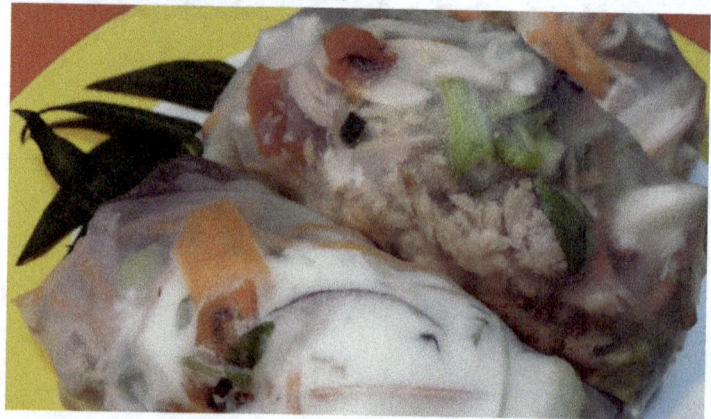

21. Tuna, Fukujinsuke, coriander, fennel

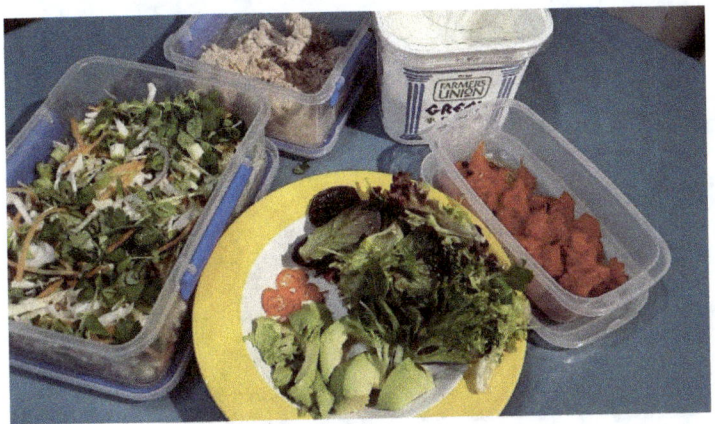

- 3 rice paper rounds
- 150g tinned tuna in springwater, drained
- Greek yoghurt
- ¼ avocado
- Fukujinzuke (Japanese sweet pickled vegetables)
- ABC very hot chilli sauce
- Mixed mesculin salad greens
- Crunchy Coleslaw veg, dry
- Chopped shallots
- Snow pea sprouts
- Fresh herbs (coriander, fennel)

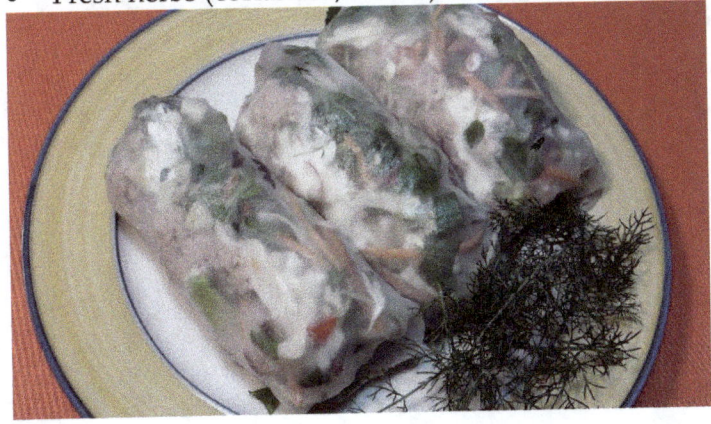

22. Tuna, sambal, Viet mint

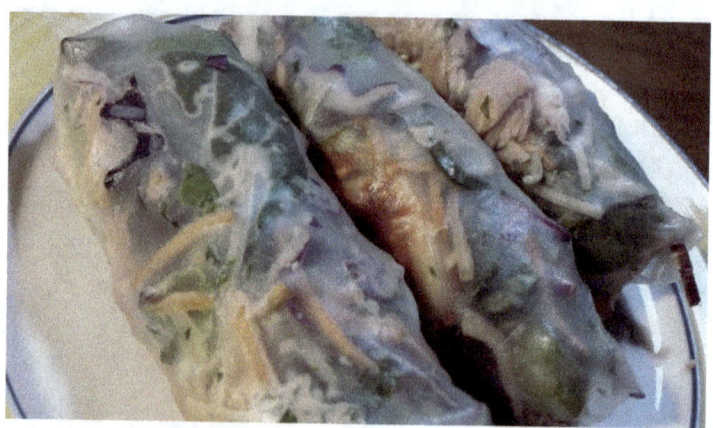

- 3 rice paper rounds
- 150g tinned tuna in springwater, drained
- Greek yoghurt
- ¼ avocado
- Conimex Sambal Oelek chilli paste
- Mixed lettuce
- Mixed coleslaw veg, with dressing
- Fresh Vietnamese mint

23. Tuna, Trident, kaleslaw, Oakleaf

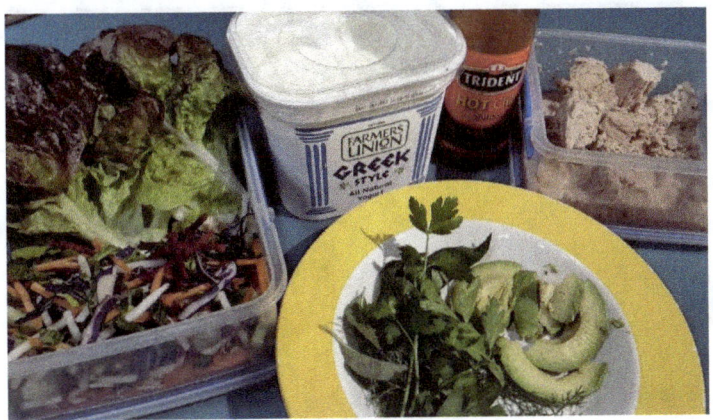

- 3 rice paper rounds
- 150g tinned tuna in springwater, drained
- Greek yoghurt
- ¼ avocado
- Trident Hot Chilli Sauce
- Kaleslaw (dry)
- Oakleaf lettuce
- Fresh herbs (Vietnamese mint, parsley, fennel)

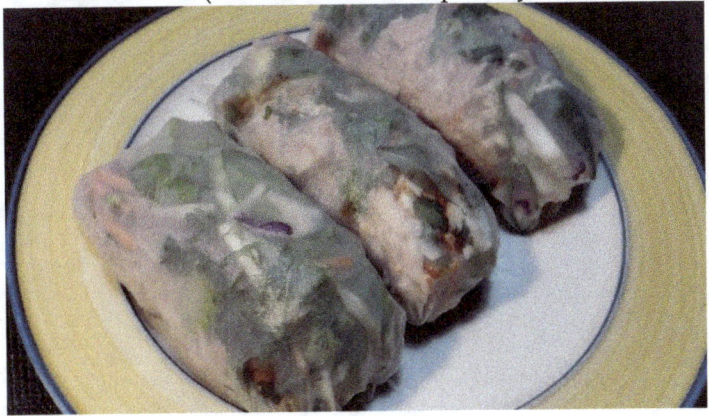

24. Tuna, chilli, Viet mint, fennel

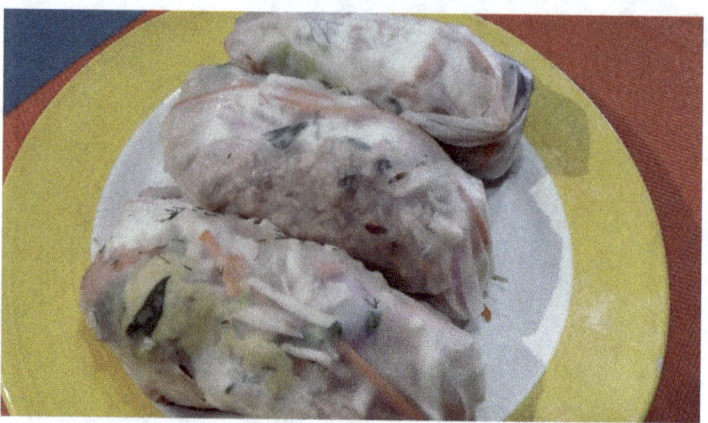

- 3 rice paper rounds
- 150g tinned tuna in springwater, drained
- Greek yoghurt
- ¼ avocado
- Teaspoon fresh chopped red chilli
- Mixed lettuce
- Crunchy Coleslaw veg, dry
- Fresh herbs (Vietnamese mint, fennel)

25. Tuna, chilli, lime, coriander

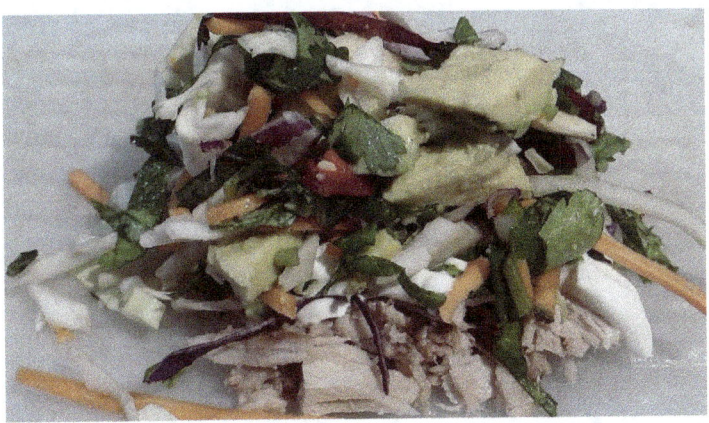

- 3 rice paper rounds
- 150g tinned tuna in springwater, drained
- Greek yoghurt
- ¼ avocado
- Teaspoon fresh chopped red chilli
- Lime juice
- Mixed kale/coleslaw
- Fresh coriander

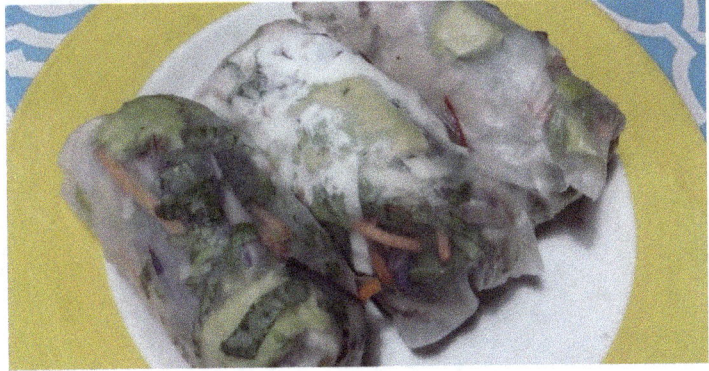

26. Tuna, spicy kaleslaw, coriander

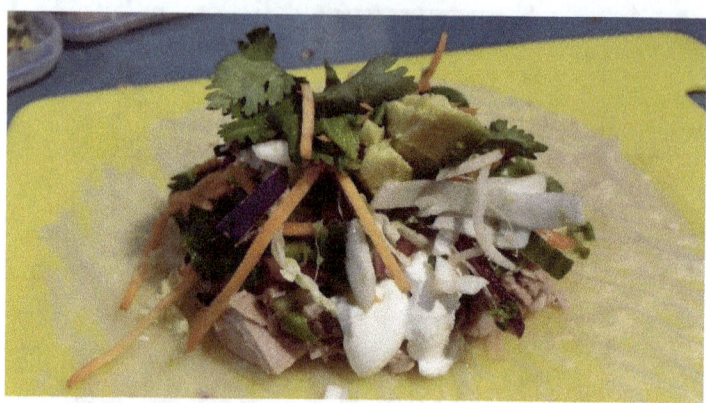

- 3 rice paper rounds
- 150g tinned tuna in springwater, drained
- Greek yoghurt
- ¼ avocado
- Mixed kale/coleslaw, with spicy dressing
- Baby lettuce leaves
- Fresh coriander

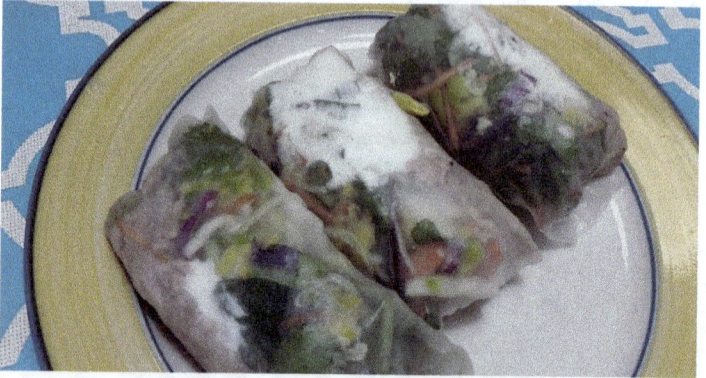

27. Tuna, jalapenos, kaleslaw, alfalfa

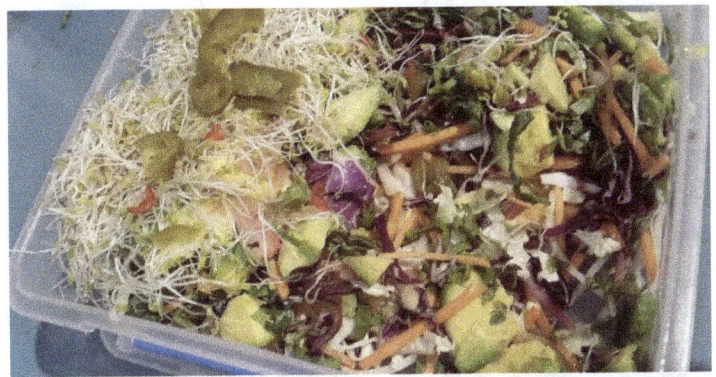

- 3 rice paper rounds
- 150g tinned tuna in springwater, drained
- Greek yoghurt
- ¼ avocado
- Pickled jalapenos, chopped
- Red chilli, chopped
- Mixed kale/coleslaw
- Baby lettuce leaves
- Alfalfa sprouts

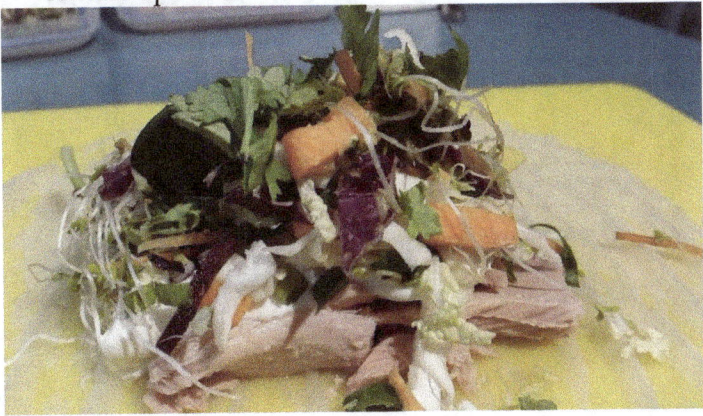

28. Tuna, Trident, coleslaw

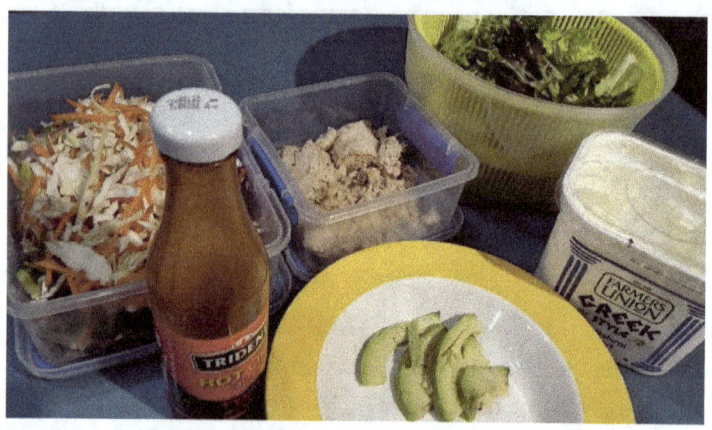

- 3 rice paper rounds
- 150g tinned tuna in springwater, drained
- Greek yoghurt
- ¼ avocado
- Trident Hot Chilli Sauce
- Crunchy Coleslaw Salad kit (dry)
- Oakleaf lettuce

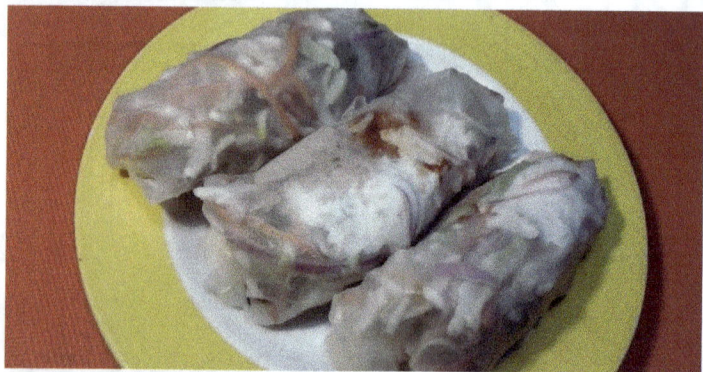

29. Tuna, green avo salad, vinegar

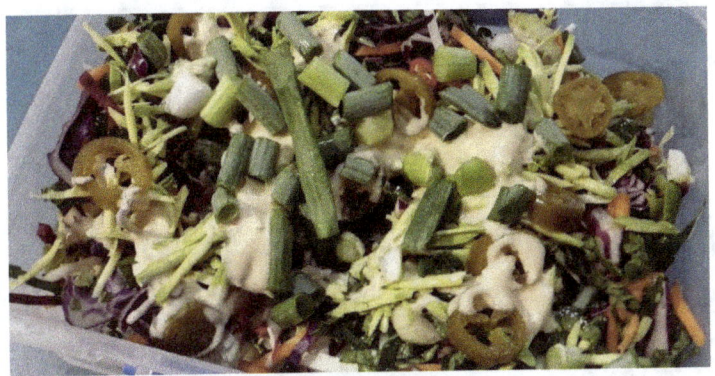

- 3 rice paper rounds
- 150g tinned tuna in springwater, drained
- Greek yoghurt
- ½ unripe avocado, finely grated
- Splash of apple cider vinegar
- Pickled jalapenos, chopped
- Fresh schallot, chopped
- Teaspoon fresh red chili, chopped
- Mixed kale/coleslaw, with spicy dressing
- Baby lettuce leaves

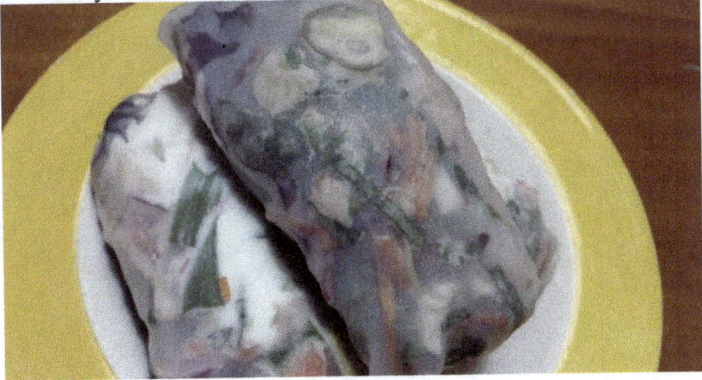

30. Tuna, green avo salad, fennel

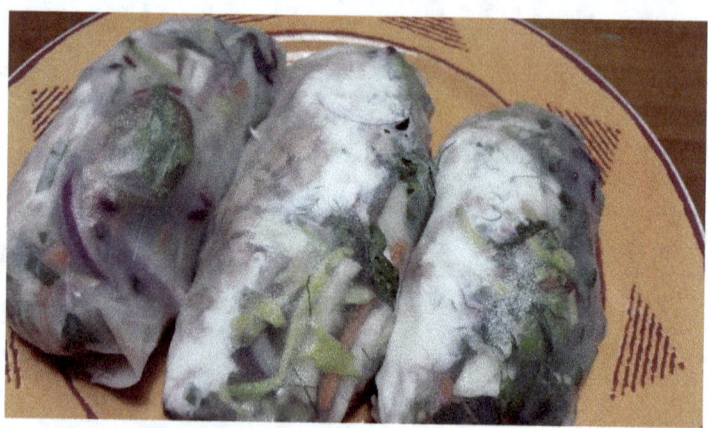

- 3 rice paper rounds
- 150g tinned tuna in springwater, drained
- Greek yoghurt
- ½ unripe avocado, finely grated
- Splash of apple cider vinegar
- Pickled jalapenos, chopped
- Fresh schallot, chopped
- Teaspoon fresh red chili, chopped
- Mixed kale/coleslaw, with spicy dressing
- Baby lettuce leaves
- Baby grated fennel bulb plus green fronds

TUNA ROLLS without yoghurt

When not using yoghurt in a recipe, you can recreate a smooth and creamy texture by doubling the amount of avocado from ¼ to ½, or add a drizzle of salad dressing… but don't do it too often if you're trying to lose weight.

31. Tuna, spicy Thai mizuna, sambal

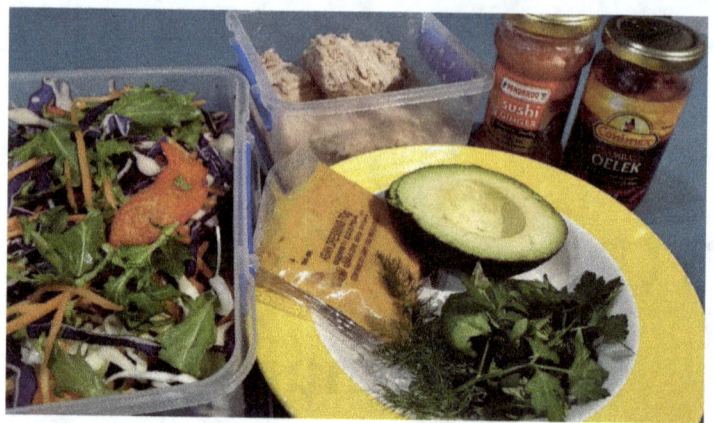

There is no yoghurt in this recipe, so we use the spicy orange-coloured dressing from the Crunchy Coleslaw Salad Kit. Do this for flavour, not weight loss, but it makes for a delicious variation when in 'weight maintenance' mode.

I can eat this combination over and over. The salad is crunchy, chili is hot, ginger is sweet, dressing is tangy. Perfect balance. The Asian herbs are the key to sensational flavour. Enjoy!

- 3 rice paper rounds
- 150g tinned tuna in springwater, drained
- ½ avocado
- Teaspoon of Conimex Sambal Oelek
- Pandaroo Sushi Ginger
- Mixed kaleslaw/Thai mizuna salad kit
- Fresh herbs (fennel, Thai basil, parsley, Viet mint)
- Spicy dressing from the Crunchy Coleslaw Kit

32. Tuna, chilli, mizuna, Caesar

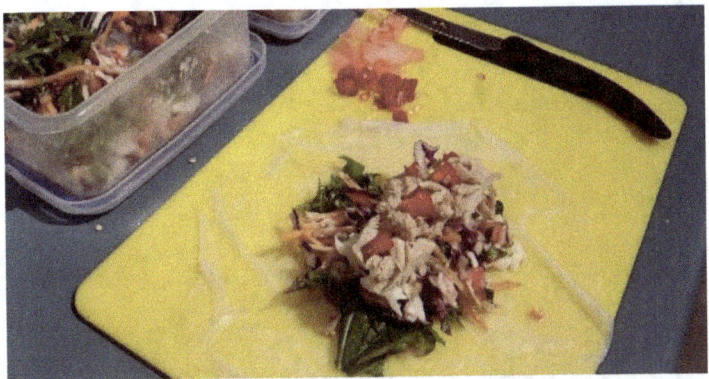

- 3 rice paper rounds
- 150g tinned tuna in springwater, drained
- A few strips of Pandaroo Sushi Ginger
- Fresh red chilli, chopped
- Cup of mixed coleslaw/Thai mizuna salad kit (dry)
- Caesar dressing

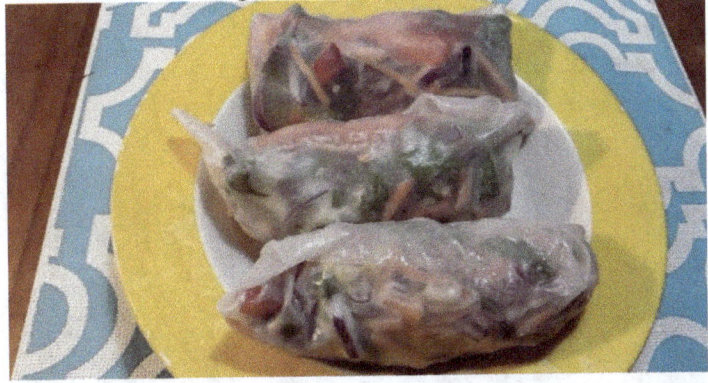

33. Tuna, kale, herbs, Chang's

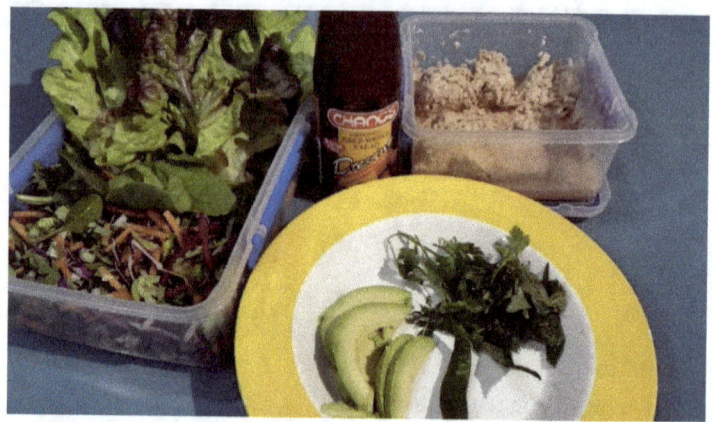

- 3 rice paper rounds
- 150g tinned tuna in springwater, drained
- ½ avocado
- Fresh green chilli, chopped
- Kaleslaw (dry)
- Baby leaf salad and beetroot salad
- Oakleaf lettuce
- Fresh herbs (Vietnamese mint, parsley, fennel)
- Chang's Oriental Fried Noodle Dipping Sauce

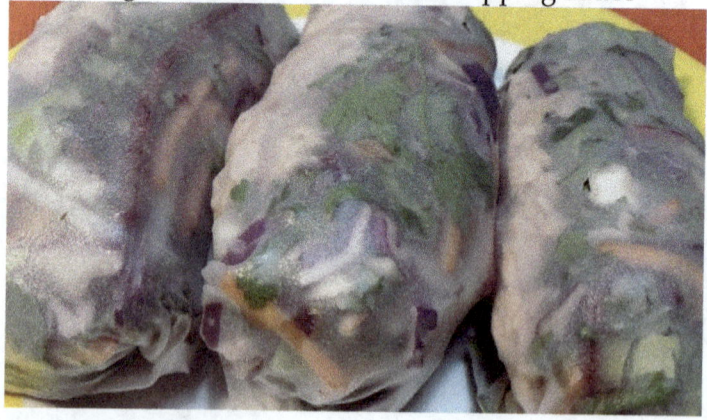

34. Tuna, spicy vinegar, Viet mint

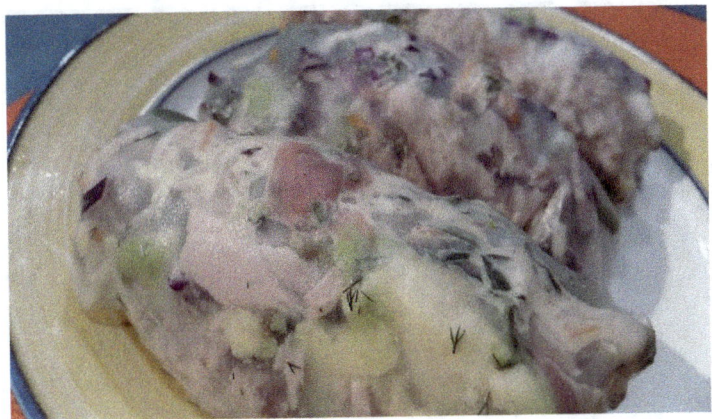

- 3 rice paper rounds
- 150g tinned tuna in springwater, drained
- ½ avocado
- Dash of vinegar from jar of jalapenos
- Pandaroo Sushi Ginger
- Mixed baby lettuce leaves
- Mixed coleslaw, with dressing
- Fresh herbs (Vietnamese mint, fennel)

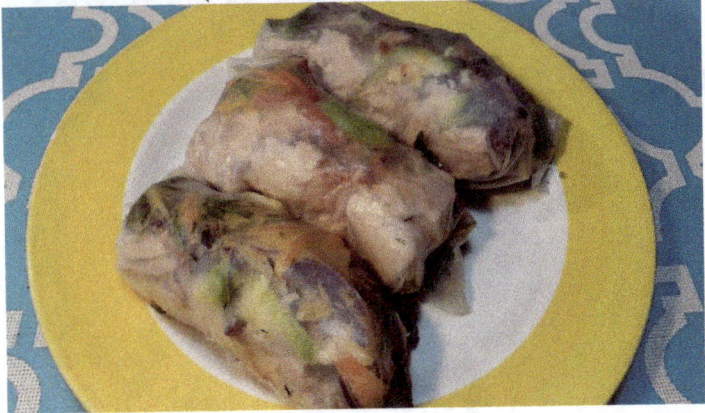

35. Tuna, lime, sambal, Thai mizuna

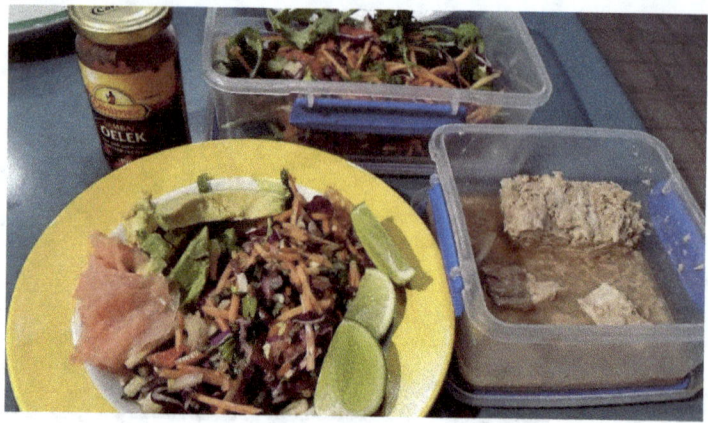

- 3 rice paper rounds
- 150g tinned tuna in springwater, drained
- ½ avocado
- Pandaroo Sushi Ginger
- Teaspoon of Conimex Sambal Oelek
- Lime juice
- Mixed kaleslaw/Thai mizuna salad kit

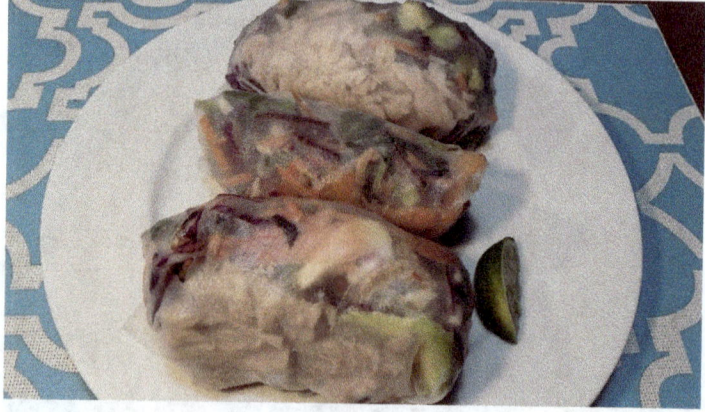

36. Tuna, pickled onion, coriander

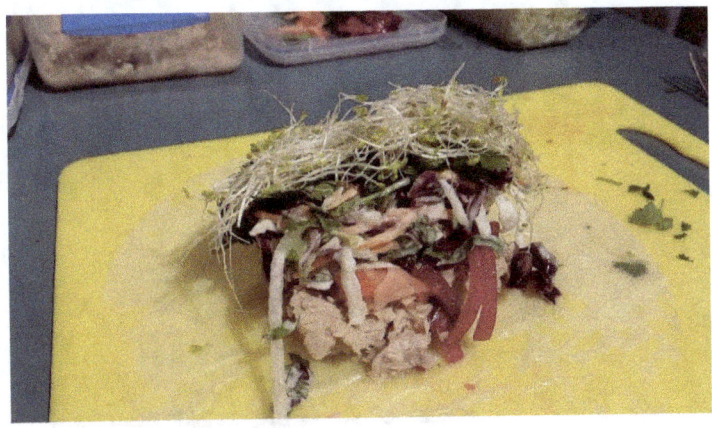

- 3 rice paper rounds
- 150g tinned tuna in springwater, drained
- Pandaroo Sushi Ginger
- Pickled red chilli, chopped
- Pickled onion, sliced
- Mix coleslaw/kaleslaw, with dressing
- Fresh coriander
- Alfalfa sprouts

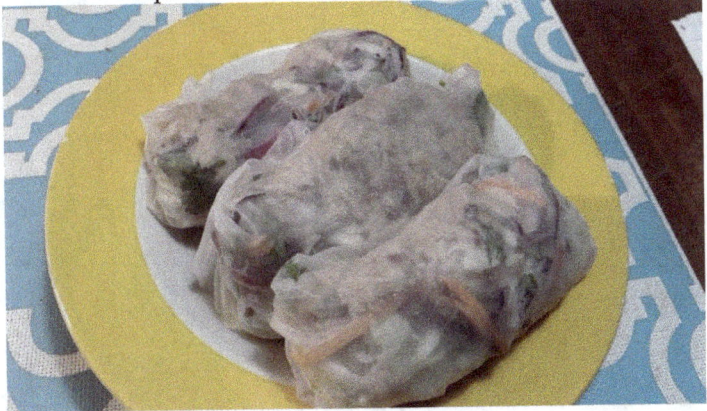

37. Tuna, onion, alfalfa, Chang's

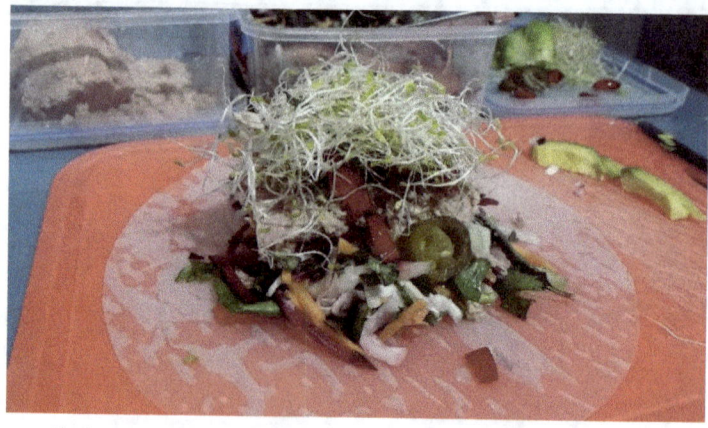

- 3 rice paper rounds
- 150g tinned tuna in springwater, drained
- ½ avocado
- Pickled jalapenos, sliced
- Fresh red onion, sliced
- Fresh red chilli, chopped
- Mixed coleslaw/kaleslaw
- Baby cos lettuce
- Alfalfa sprouts
- Fresh Vietnamese mint
- Chang's Fried Noodle Dipping Sauce

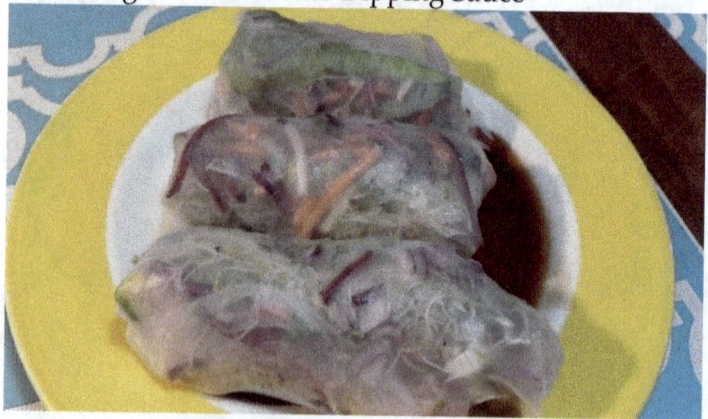

38. Tuna, jalapenos, coleslaw, fennel

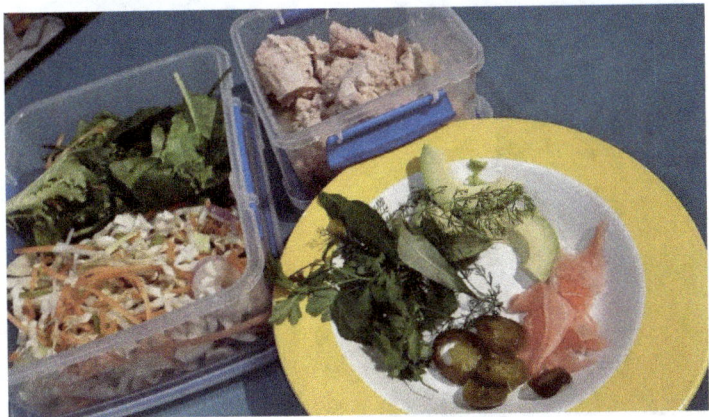

- 3 rice paper rolls
- 150g tinned tuna in springwater, drained
- ½ avocado
- Pandaroo Sushi Ginger
- Pickled jalapenos, sliced
- Coleslaw
- Baby leaf salad
- Fresh herbs (Vietnamese mint, parsley, fennel)

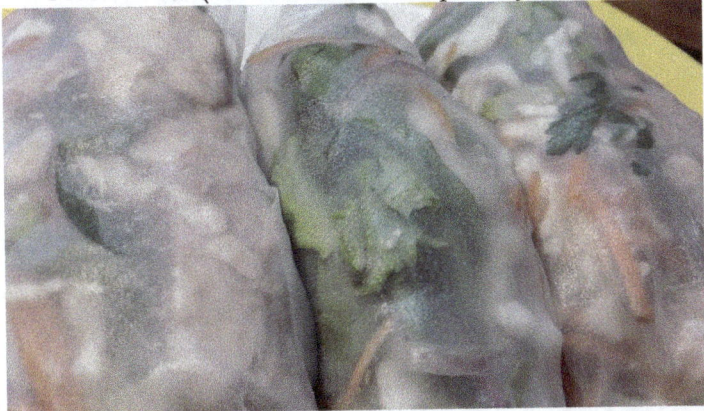

39. Tuna, baby leaf, Trident, Thai basil

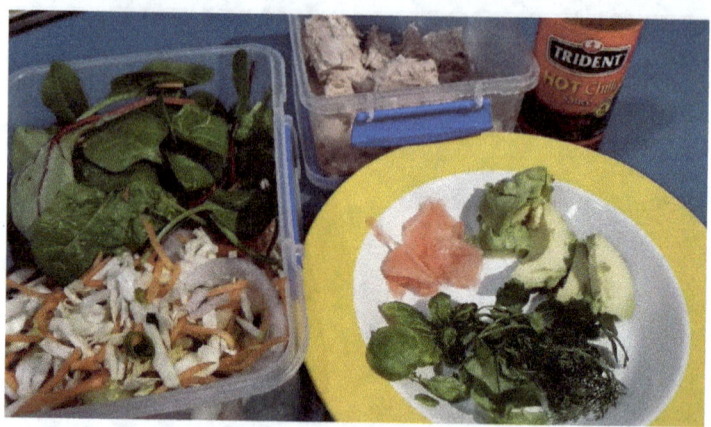

- 3 rice paper rolls
- 150g tinned tuna in springwater, drained
- ½ avocado
- Pandaroo Sushi Ginger
- Trident Hot Chilli Sauce
- Coleslaw
- Baby leaf salad with shredded beetroot
- Fresh herbs (Thai basil, parsley, fennel)

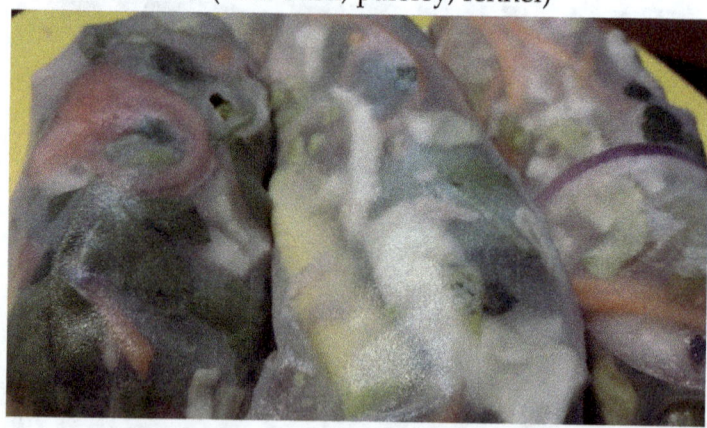

40. Tuna, silverbeet, pineapple, lemon

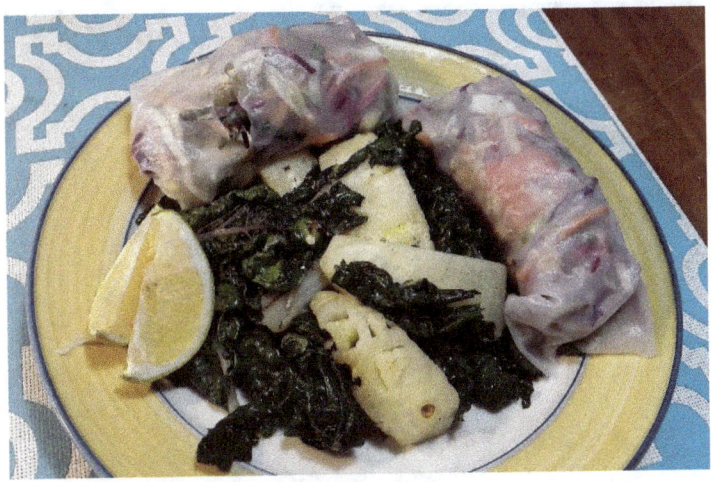

- 3 rice paper rolls
- 150g tinned tuna in springwater, drained
- ½ avocado
- Pandaroo Sushi Ginger
- Kaleslaw with dressing
- Serve rolls on a bed of pan-seared silverbeet, pineapple, lemon juice

41. Tuna, fennel root, bean sprouts

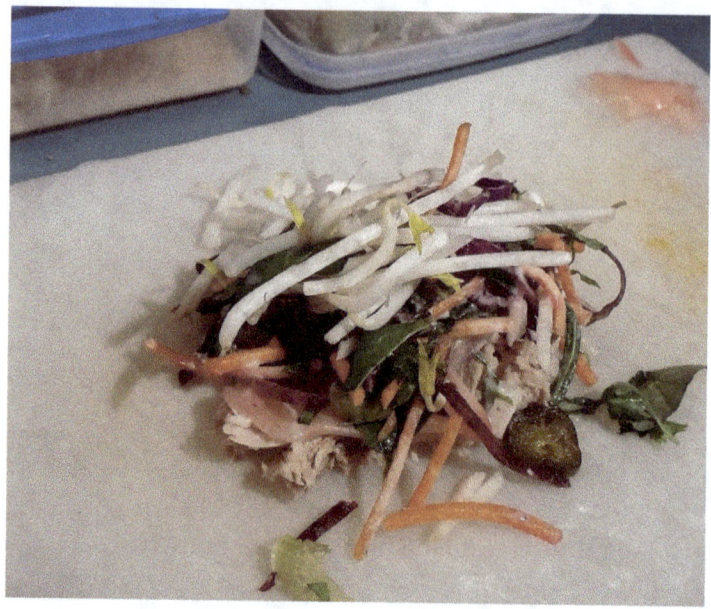

- 3 rice paper rolls
- 150g tinned tuna in springwater, drained
- Pandaroo Sushi Ginger
- Kaleslaw with dressing
- Grated fennel root (aniseed flavour)
- Fresh herbs (Vietnamese mint, coriander)
- Bean sprouts

42. Tuna, fennel root, lime, coriander

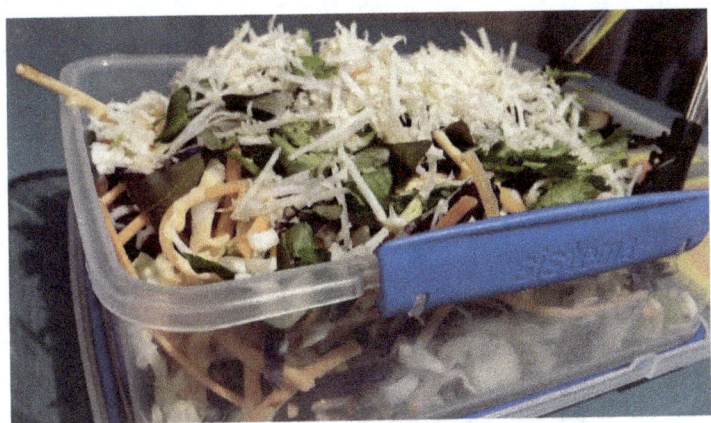

- 3 rice paper rolls
- 150g tinned tuna in springwater, drained
- ½ avocado
- Pandaroo Sushi Ginger
- Southern Style coleslaw mix
- Grated fennel root
- Fresh coriander
- Lime juice

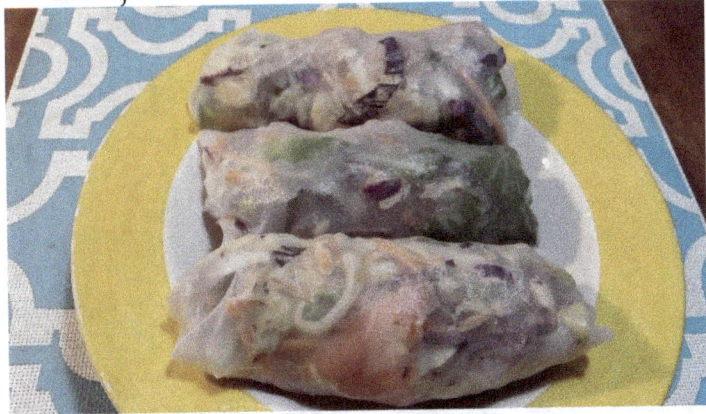

43. Tuna, sauerkraut, kale, beets

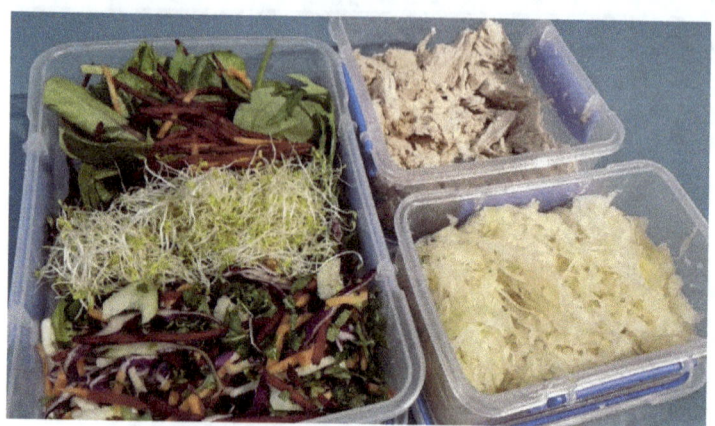

- 3 rice paper rounds
- 150g tinned tuna in springwater, drained
- ½ avocado
- Sauerkraut
- Caesar or Ranch Dressing
- Baby leaf salad
- Mixed coleslaw/kaleslaw
- Alfalfa sprouts

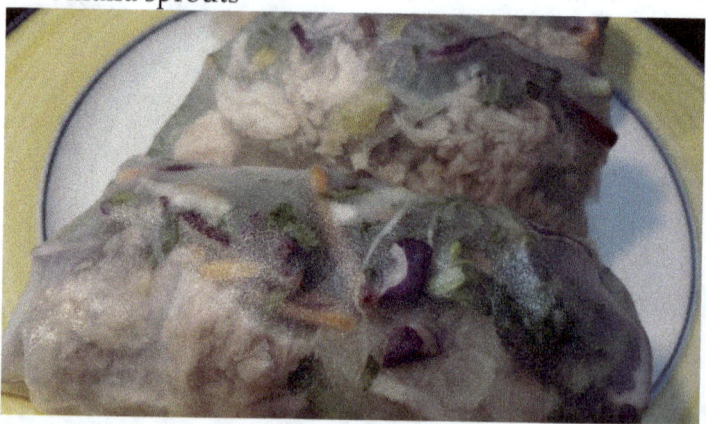

44. Tuna, tahini, jalapenos, mint

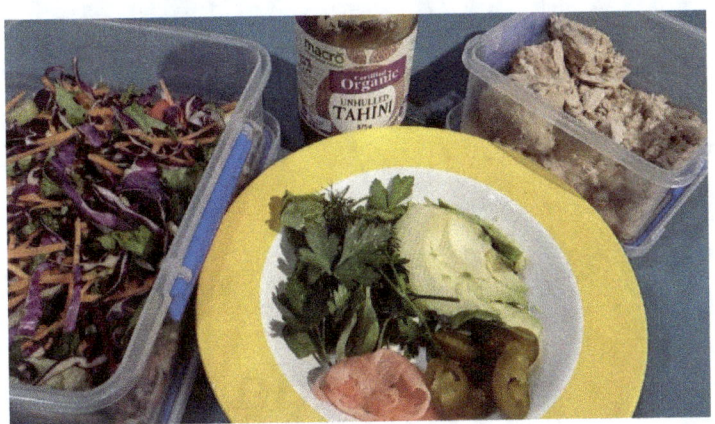

- 3 rice paper rounds
- 150g tinned tuna in springwater, drained
- ½ avocado
- 1 dessertspoon of tahini paste
- Pandaroo Sushi Ginger
- Pickled jalapenos, sliced
- Mixed kaleslaw/Thai Mizuna Salad kit
- Fresh herbs (Thai Basil, parsley, Vietnamese mint)

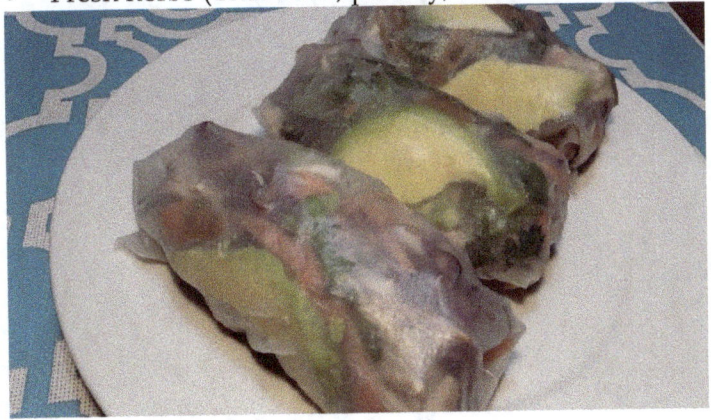

TUNA ROLLS without avocado

Avocado adds unsaturated fats and a creamy textural element, but it can slow your weight loss if eaten every day.

But a delicious flavour profile can be easily achieved by the clever use of Greek yoghurt, condiments, and the occasional salad dressing.

45. Tuna, Viet mint, mixed slaw

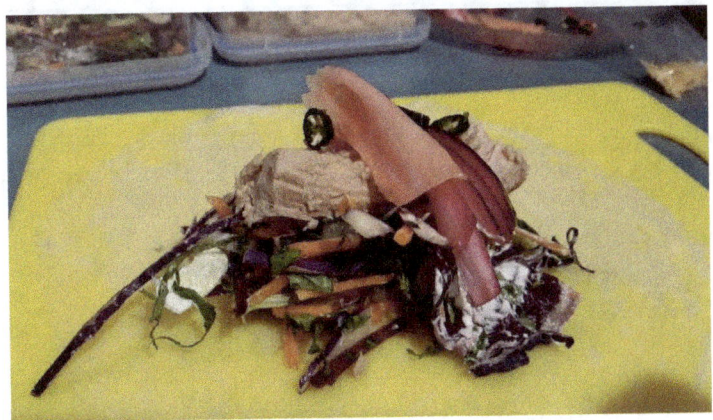

- 3 rice paper rounds
- 150g tinned tuna in springwater, drained
- Greek yoghurt
- Pandaroo Sushi Ginger
- Southern Style coleslaw/kaleslaw (dry)
- Fresh herbs (parsley, Vietnamese mint)
- Sprinkle with fried onion flakes
- Poonsin Vietnamese Spring Roll Dipping Sauce

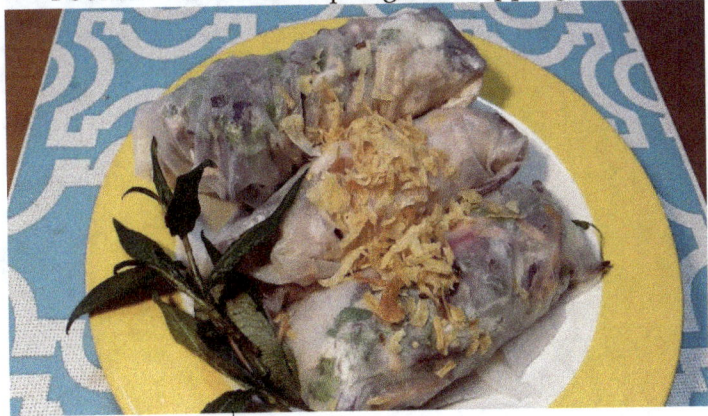

46. Tuna, Thai mizuna, herbs

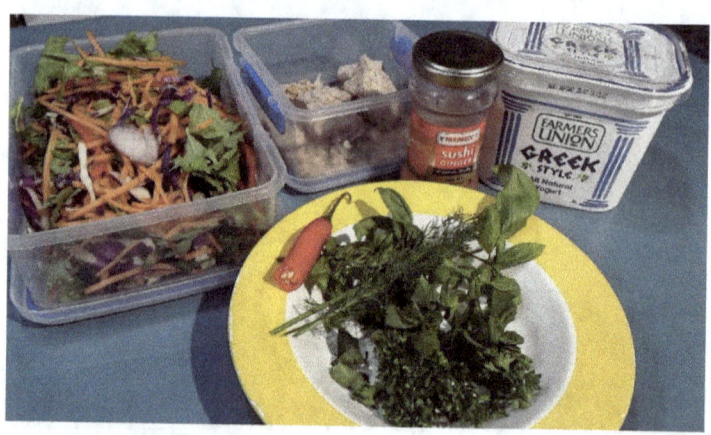

- 3 rice paper rounds
- 150g tinned tuna in springwater, drained
- Greek yoghurt
- Pandaroo Sushi Ginger
- Mild chilli, chopped
- Thai mizuna salad kit (dry)
- Fresh herbs (Viet mint, Thai basil, parsley, fennel)

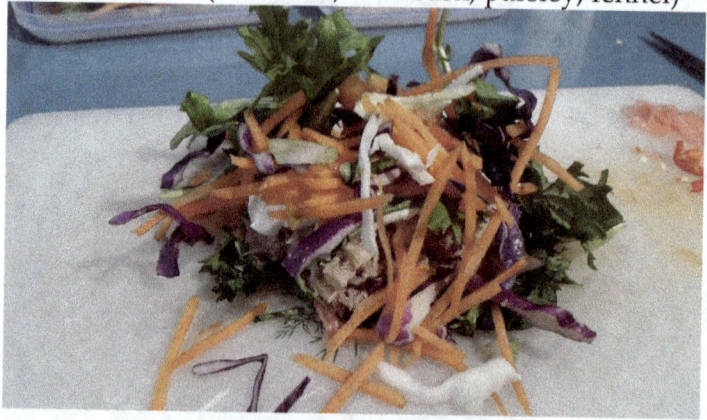

47. Tuna, kale, alfalfa

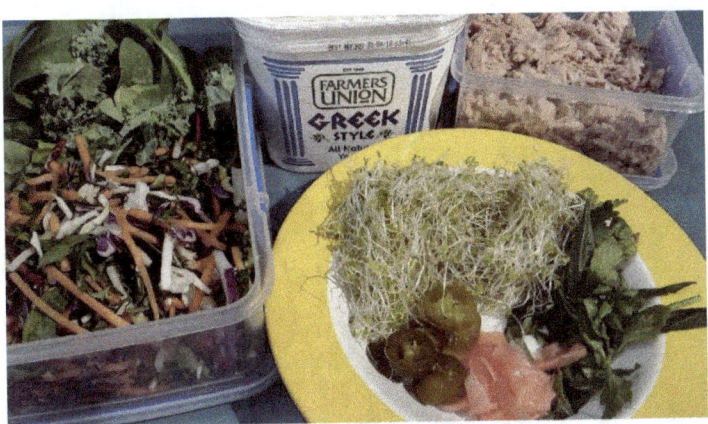

- 3 rice paper rounds
- 150g tinned tuna in springwater, drained
- Greek yoghurt
- Pandaroo Sushi Ginger
- Pickled jalapenos, sliced
- Baby spinach and kale salad greens
- Mixed coleslaw/kaleslaw
- Fresh herbs (Vietnamese mint, parsley, Thai basil)
- Alfalfa sprouts
- Chang's Oriental Noodle Salad dressing

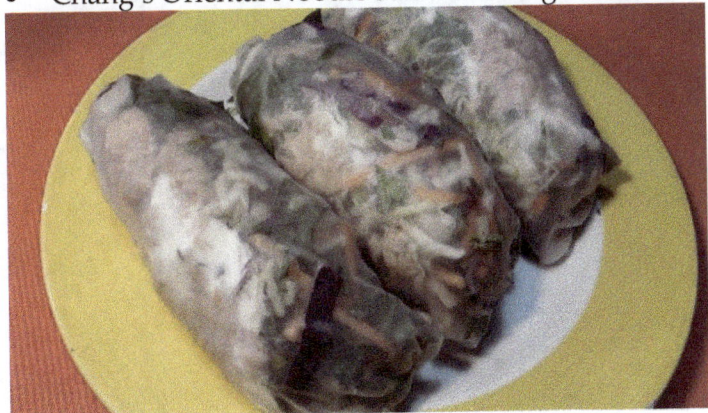

48. Tuna, Trident, onion, dill

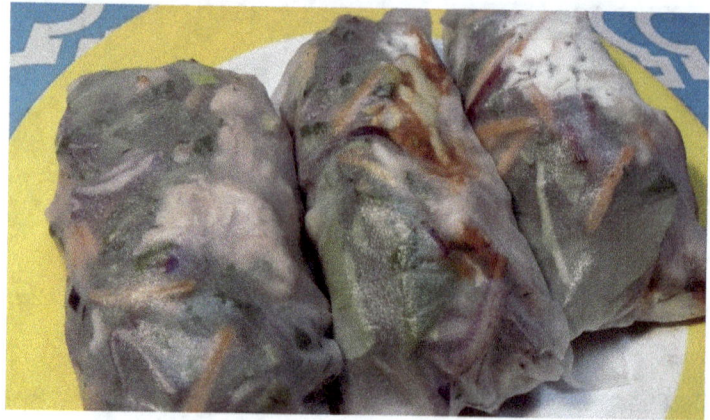

- 3 rice paper rounds
- 150g tinned tuna in springwater, drained
- Greek yoghurt
- Trident Hot Chilli Sauce
- Kaleslaw (dry)
- Baby Leaf and Shredded Beetroot Salad
- A few slices of red onion
- Fresh dill

49. Tuna, chilli, onion, mixed slaw

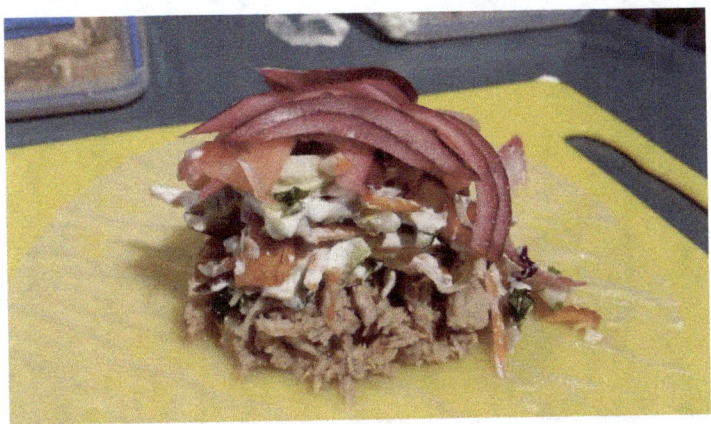

- 3 rice paper rounds
- 150g tinned tuna in springwater, drained
- Greek yoghurt
- Pandaroo Sushi Ginger
- Pickled red onion, sliced
- Fresh red chilli, chopped
- Mixed coleslaw/kaleslaw (dry)
- Fresh Thai basil (tastes better than Italian basil)

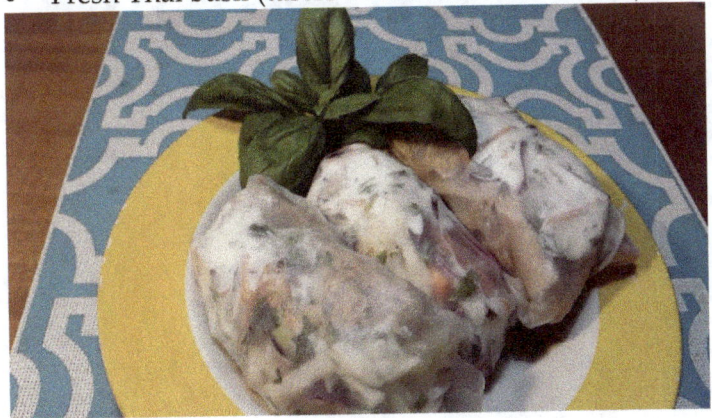

50. Tuna, kaleslaw, Chang's sauce

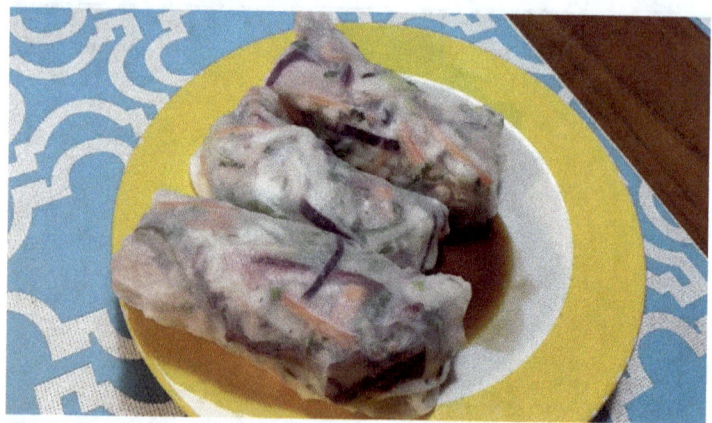

- 3 rice paper rounds
- 150g tinned tuna in springwater, drained
- Greek yoghurt
- Pandaroo Sushi Ginger
- Pickled jalapenos, chopped
- Mixed coleslaw/kaleslaw
- Chang's Fried Noodle Dipping Sauce

51. Tuna, grilled capsicum, pineapple

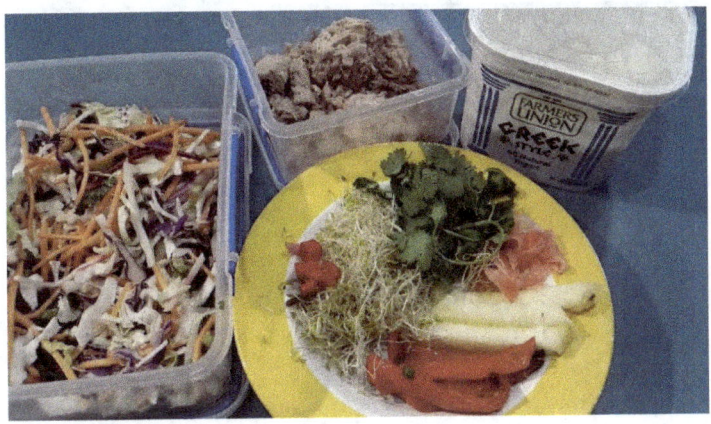

- 3 rice paper rounds
- 150g tinned tuna in springwater, drained
- Greek yoghurt
- Pandaroo Sushi Ginger
- Pickled red chilli, chopped
- Roasted/grilled red capsicum, sliced
- Fresh pineapple, sliced
- Mixed coleslaw
- Fresh coriander
- Alfalfa sprouts

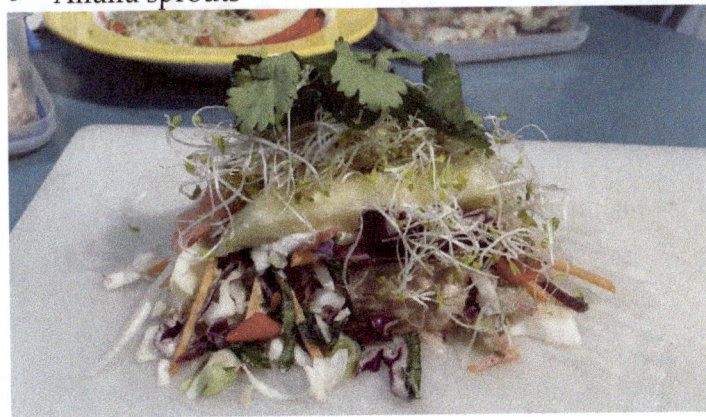

52. Tuna, tahini, beetroot, jalapenos

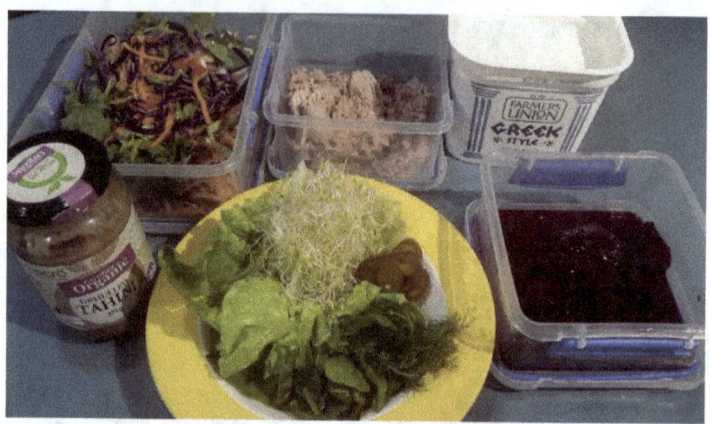

Tahini is such a welcome change, with its delicious peanut-like flavour and bitterness, offset by creamy yoghurt and spicy jalapenos. The addition of lettuce and beetroot is perfect, and the herbs punch thru once or twice for a fresh surprise. Middle-eastern fusion.

- 3 rice paper rounds
- 150g tinned tuna in springwater, drained
- Greek yoghurt
- Tahini
- Beetroot
- Pickled jalapenos, sliced
- Butter lettuce
- Alfalfa sprouts
- Mixed Thai Mizuna Salad/kaleslaw
- Fresh herbs (Thai basil, dill, Viet mint)

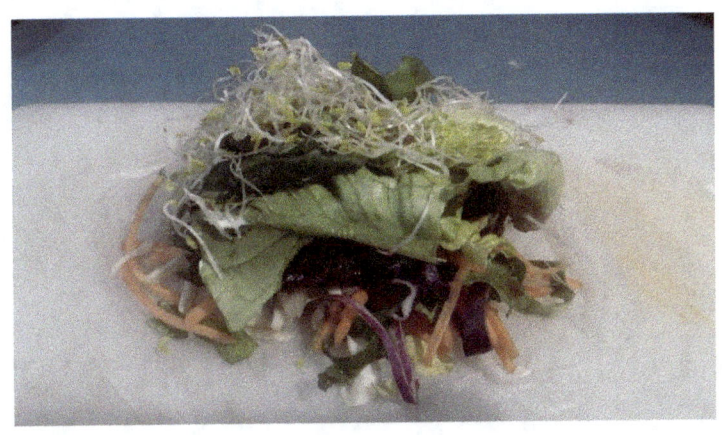

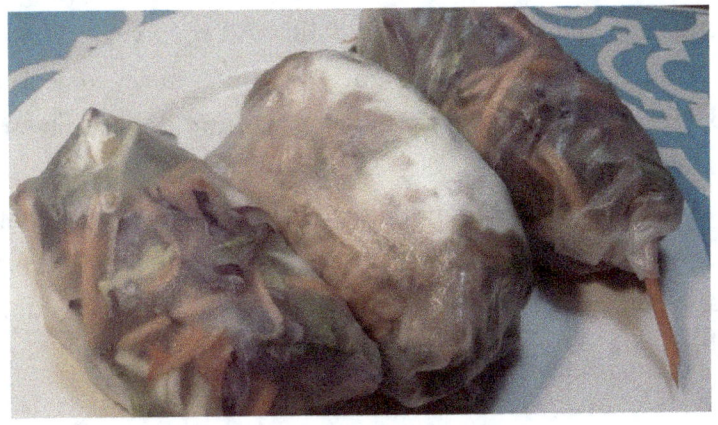

TUNA ROLLS with nori

These recipes take inspiration from Japanese sushi rolls, wrapped in sheets of nori seaweed, and filled with perfectly balanced ingredients such as tuna, avocado, pickled ginger, a spicy element such as wasabi or chilli, and crisp vegetables.

Nori seaweed is high in nutrients, but it can become tough and chewy when damp. This is why we snip it into thin strips before adding it to the inside or outside of a rice paper roll.

Greek yoghurt is not always a good accompaniment to Japanese nori, so most of these recipes are dairy-free. Hence, the creamy element is often satisfied by using more avocado, or adding another salad dressing.

53. Tuna, nori, sambal, avo, fennel

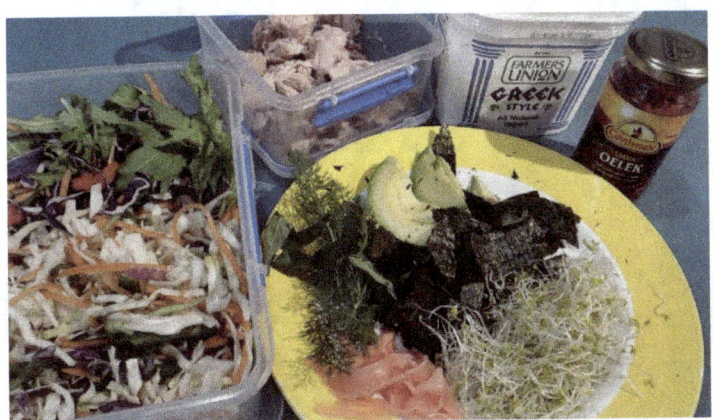

- 3 rice paper rounds
- 150g tinned tuna in springwater, drained
- Greek yoghurt
- ¼ avocado
- Lime juice
- Conimex Sambal Oelek
- Mixed coleslaw/Asian salad
- Alfalfa sprouts
- Fresh herbs (Vietnamese mint, parsley, fennel)
- ½ nori sheet, shredded

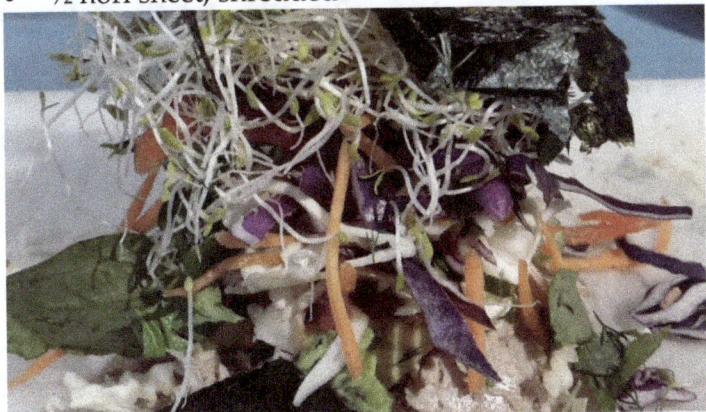

54. Tuna, nori, ginger, dill

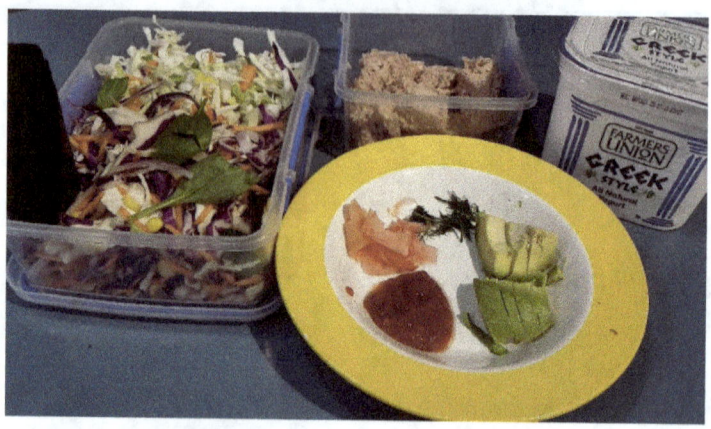

- 3 rice paper rounds
- 150g tinned tuna in springwater, drained
- Greek yoghurt
- ½ avocado
- Pandaroo Sushi Ginger
- Conimex Sambal Oelek
- Mixed coleslaw with Rainbow Coleslaw Salad kit
- Fresh dill
- Nori strips

55. Tuna, nori, chilli, onion flakes

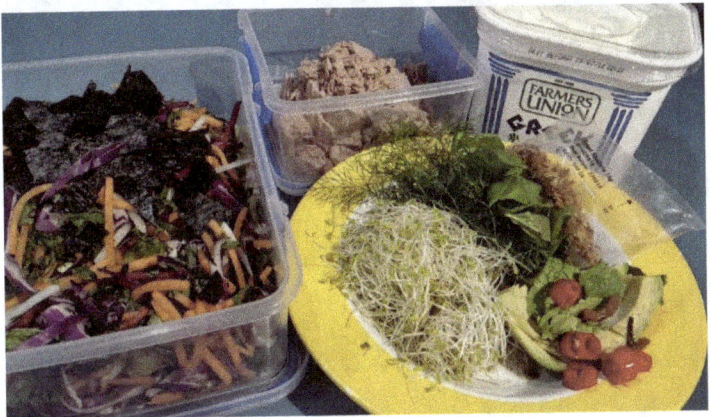

- 3 rice paper rounds
- 150g tinned John West tuna in springwater, drained
- Greek yoghurt
- ¼ avocado
- Red chilli, chopped
- Pandaroo Sushi Ginger
- Conimex Sambal Oelek
- Mixed kale/coleslaw
- Alfalfa
- Fresh herbs (fennel, Thai basil)
- Crispy onion flakes (from salad kit)
- Nori strips

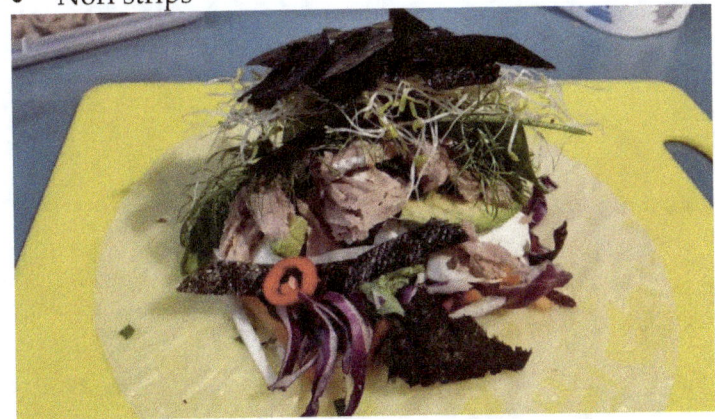

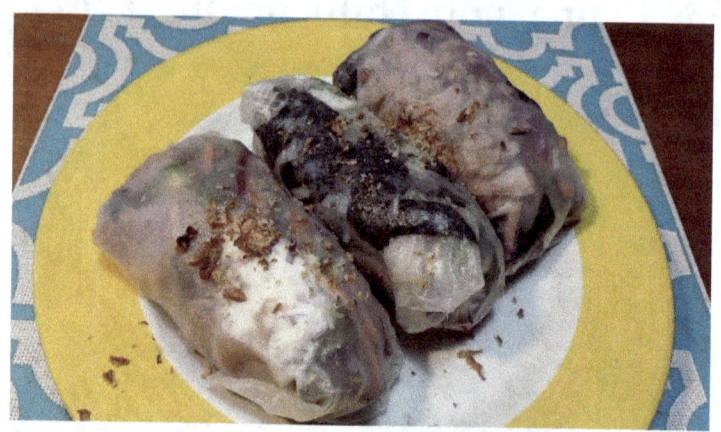

56. Tuna, nori, Viet mint, fennel

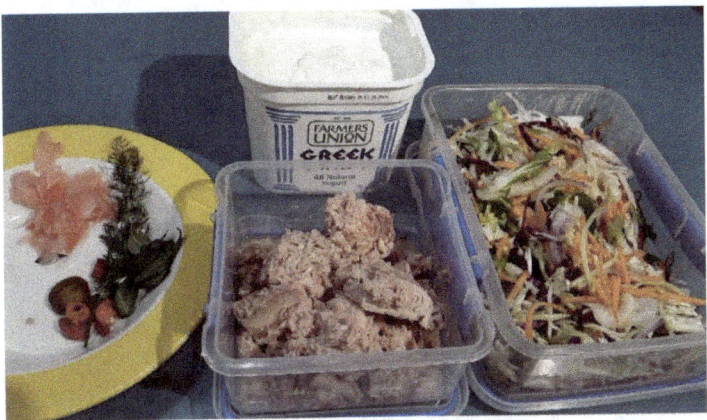

- 3 rice paper rounds
- 150g tinned tuna in springwater, drained
- Greek yoghurt
- Pandaroo Sushi Ginger
- Fresh red chilli, chopped
- Grated fennel bulb
- Mixed coleslaw (Southern, Kale, Asian)
- Fresh herbs (Vietnamese mint, fennel fronds)
- Nori strips

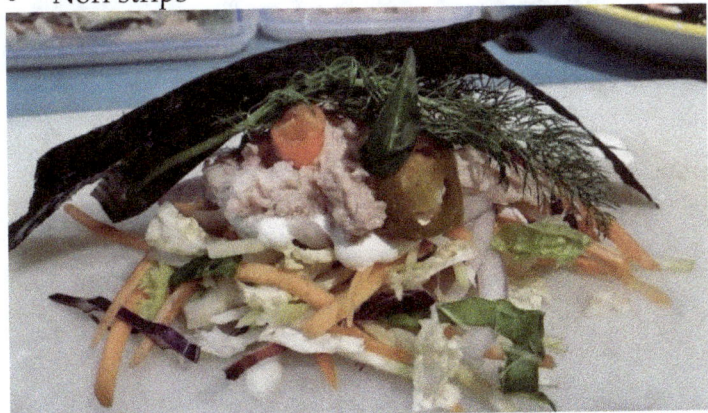

57. Tuna, nori, basil, fennel

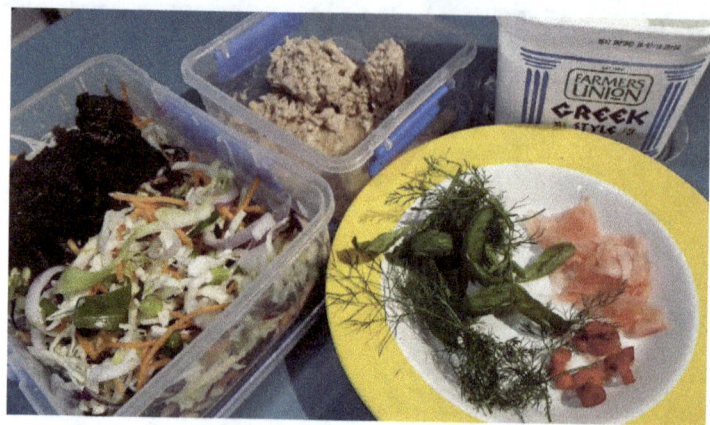

- 3 rice paper rounds
- 150g tinned tuna in springwater, drained
- Greek yoghurt
- Pandaroo Sushi Ginger
- Fresh red chilli, chopped
- Grated fennel bulb
- Coleslaw with onion
- Fresh herbs (basil, fennel) – Thai basil is better
- Nori strips

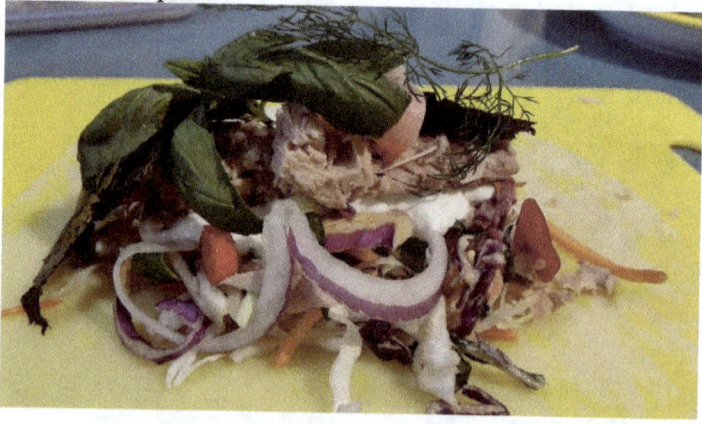

58. Tuna, nori, kaleslaw

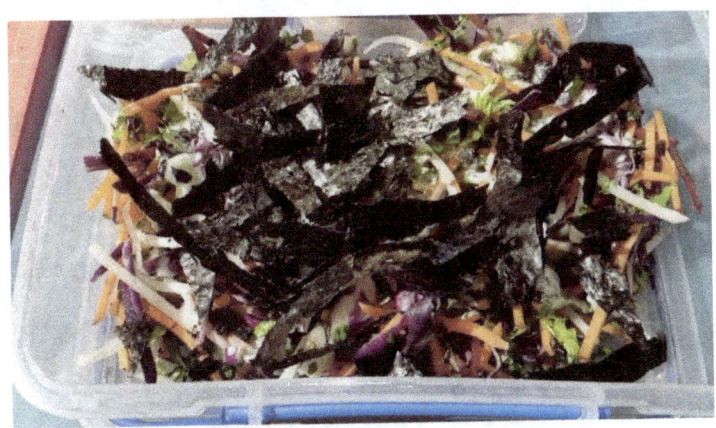

- 3 rice paper rounds
- 150g tinned tuna in springwater, drained
- ½ avocado
- Pandaroo Sushi Ginger
- Pickled jalapenos, chopped
- Pickled red chilli, chopped
- Kaleslaw with dressing
- ½ sheet Nori seaweed, snipped into thin pieces

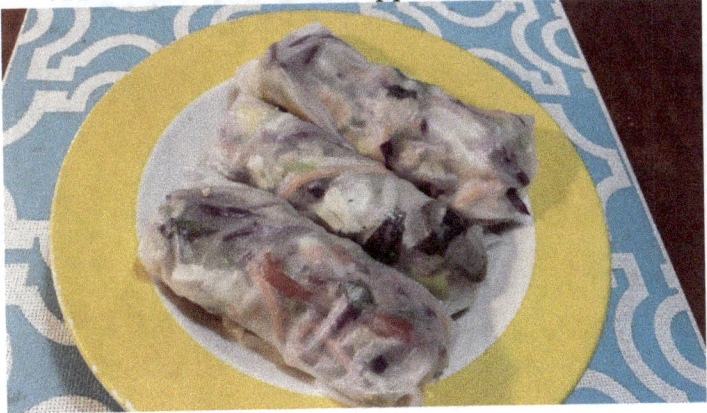

59. Tuna, nori, Trident, kaleslaw

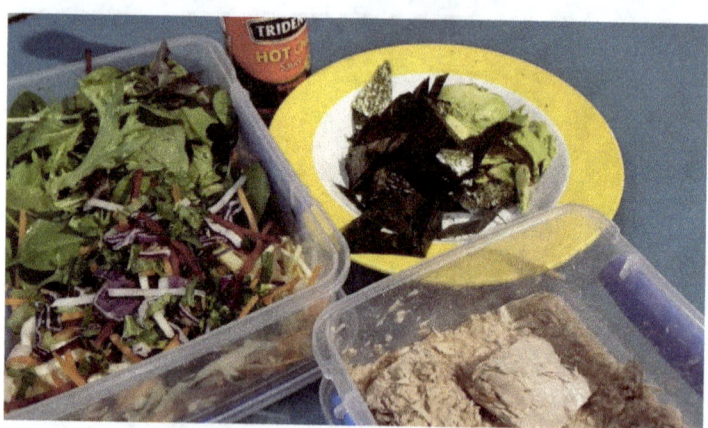

- 3 rice paper rounds
- 150g tinned tuna in springwater, drained
- ½ avocado
- Trident Hot Chilli Sauce
- Mixed coleslaw/kaleslaw
- Baby leaf and beetroot salad
- Nori strips

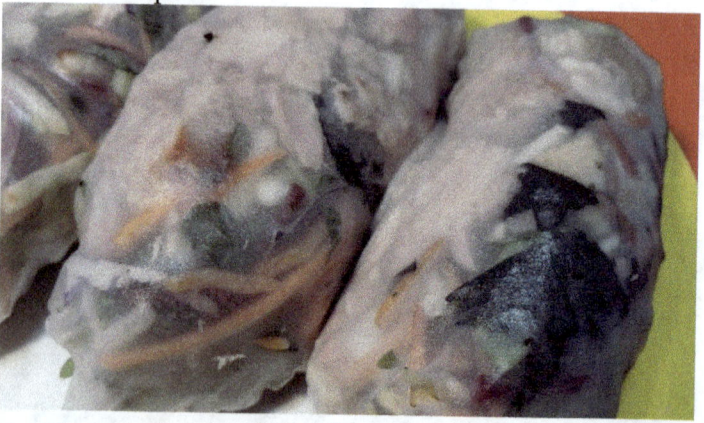

60. Tuna, nori, lime, mint

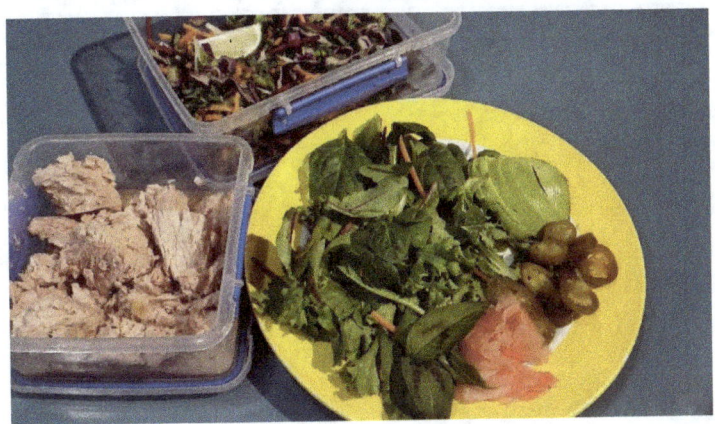

- 3 rice paper rounds
- 150g tinned tuna in springwater, drained
- ½ avocado
- Pandaroo Sushi Ginger
- Pickled jalapenos, sliced
- Lime juice
- Kaleslaw, Baby leaf salad
- Fresh Vietnamese mint
- Nori strips

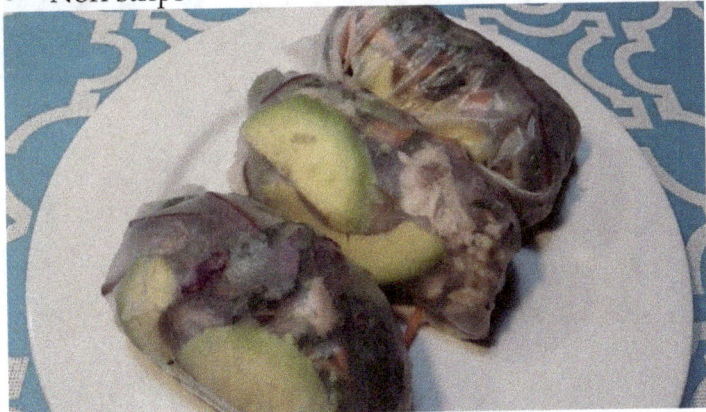

61. Tuna, nori, avo, kaleslaw

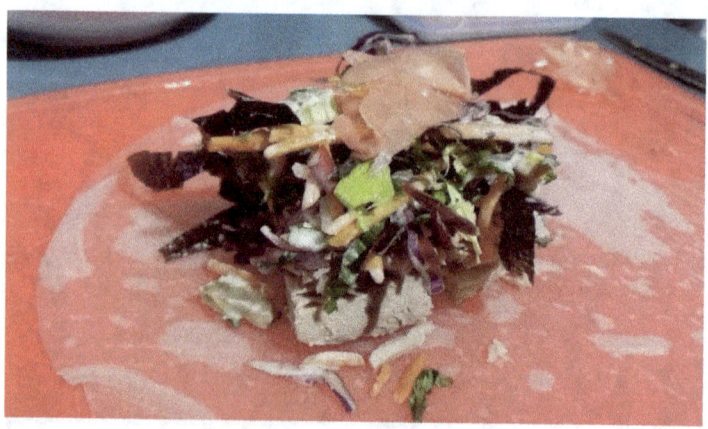

- 3 rice paper rounds
- 150g tinned tuna in springwater, drained
- ½ avocado
- Pandaroo Sushi Ginger
- Fresh red chili, chopped
- Kaleslaw with dressing
- Nori strips

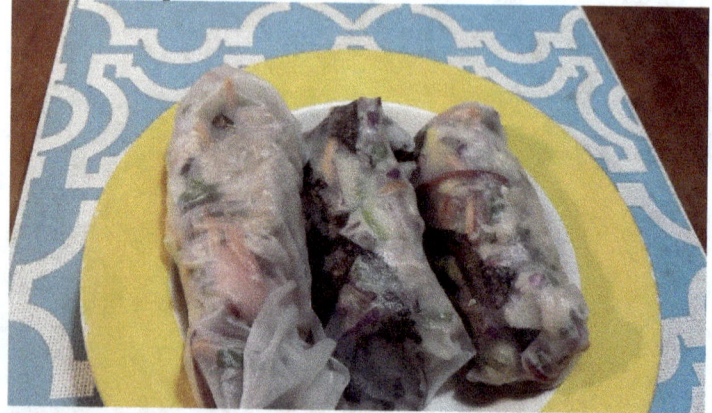

62. Tuna, nori, grilled capsicum, bean sprouts

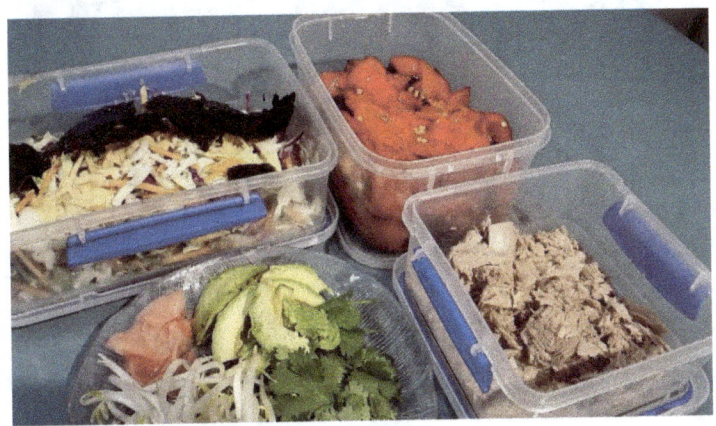

- 3 rice paper rounds
- 150g tinned tuna in springwater, drained
- ½ avocado
- Pandaroo Sushi Ginger
- Roasted red capsicum in olive oil
- Mixed coleslaw/kaleslaw with dressing
- Fresh coriander
- Bean sprouts
- Nori strips

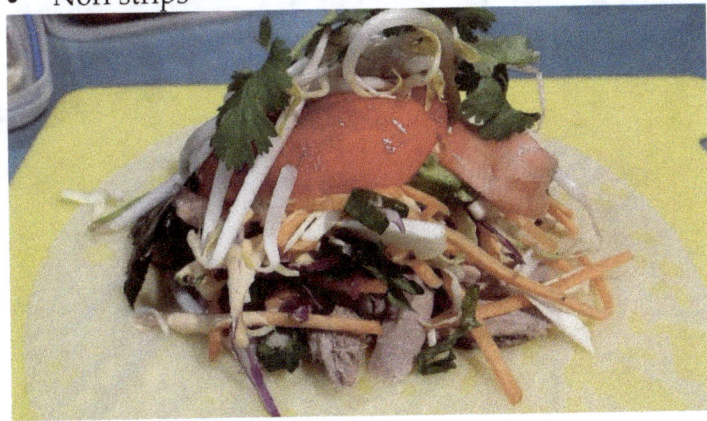

100

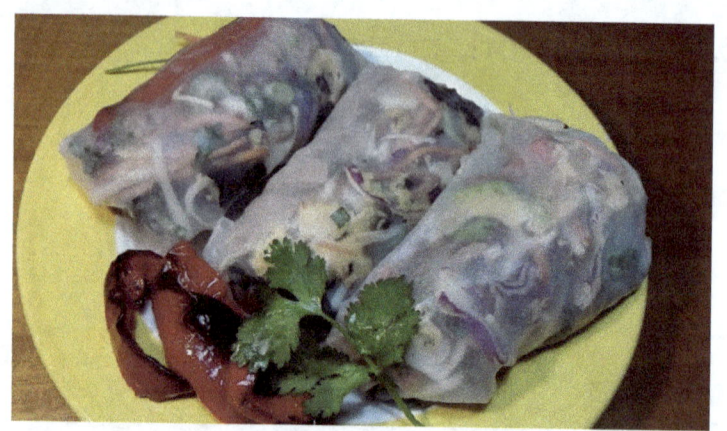

63. Tuna, nori, grilled capsicum, coriander

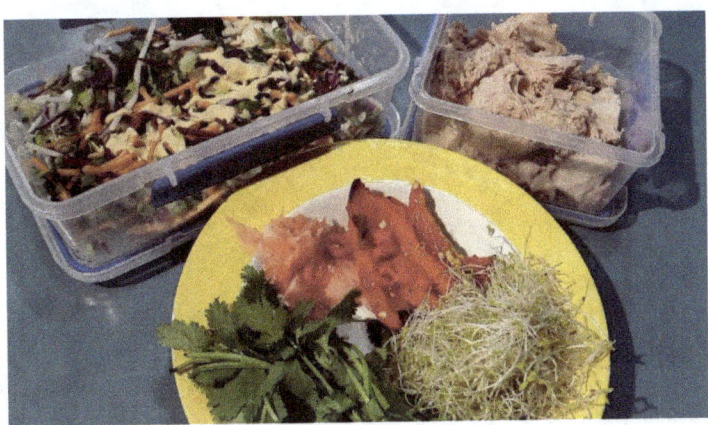

- 3 rice paper rounds
- 150g tinned tuna in springwater, drained
- Pickled red chilli, chopped
- Pandaroo Sushi Ginger
- Roasted red capsicum, sliced
- Mixed coleslaw with spicy dressing
- Fresh coriander
- Alfalfa sprouts
- Nori strips

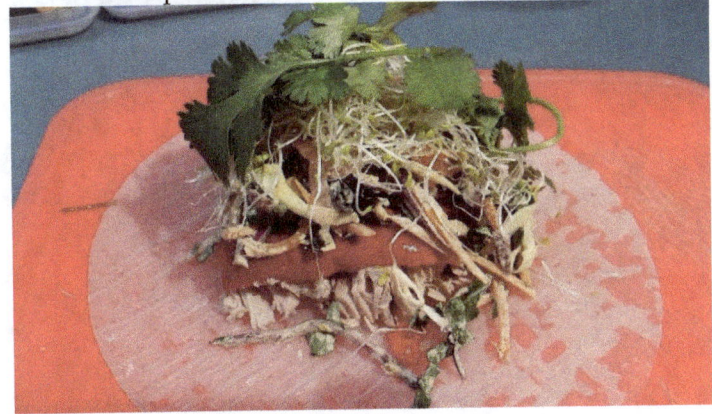

64. Tuna, nori, chilli, alfalfa

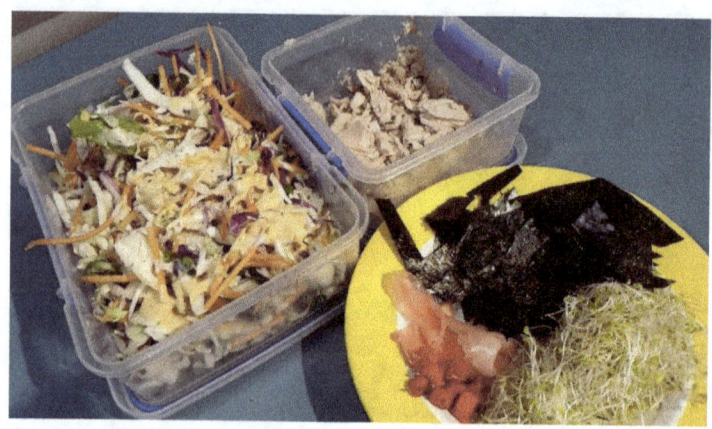

- 3 rice paper rounds
- 150g tinned tuna in springwater, drained
- Pandaroo Sushi Ginger
- Pickled red chilli, chopped
- Southern Style Coleslaw with dressing
- Alfalfa sprouts
- Nori strips

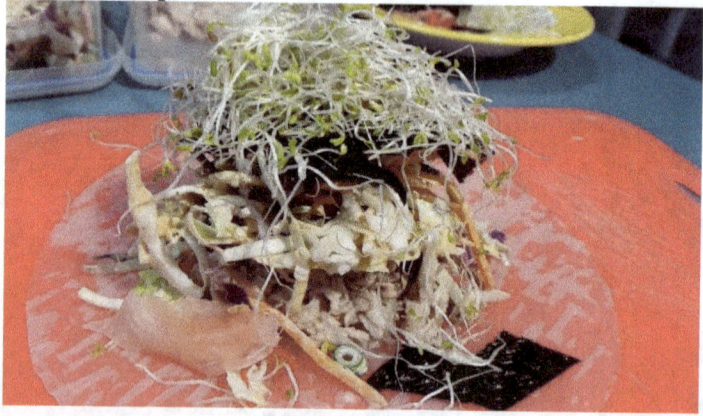

TUNA ROLLS with a hint of Mediterranean

Don't be limited in your thinking. Be daring. Be adventurous. Try incorporating other flavours and textures. Let other cultures and cuisines be your guide.

Balsamic vinegar, fresh ripe tomatoes, black olives, onion rings, basil, and crisp salads are the ingredients that make an Italian salad so special.

A few drops of Balsamic vinegar can work magic on some cheaper brands of tuna or pink salmon. It can mask any unpleasant fishy smell or taste, while adding a familiar earthy flavour of the Mediterranean.

65. Tuna, balsamic, baby leaves

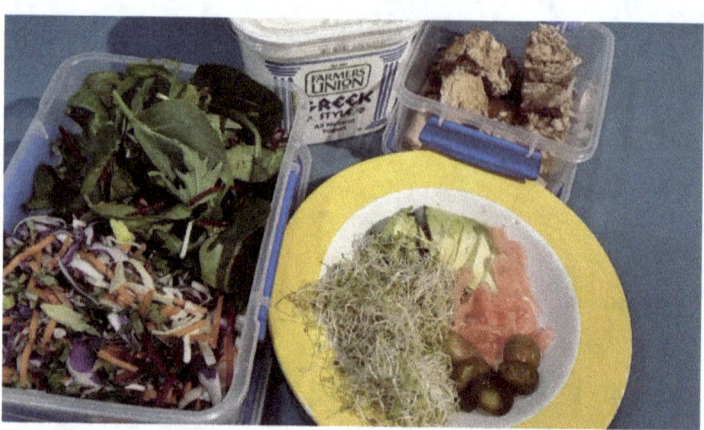

- 3 rice paper rounds
- 150g tinned tuna in springwater, drained
- Balsamic vinegar
- Greek yoghurt
- ¼ avocado
- Pandaroo Sushi Ginger
- Pickled jalapenos, sliced
- Mixed coleslaw/kaleslaw
- Baby leaf and beetroot salad
- Alfalfa sprouts

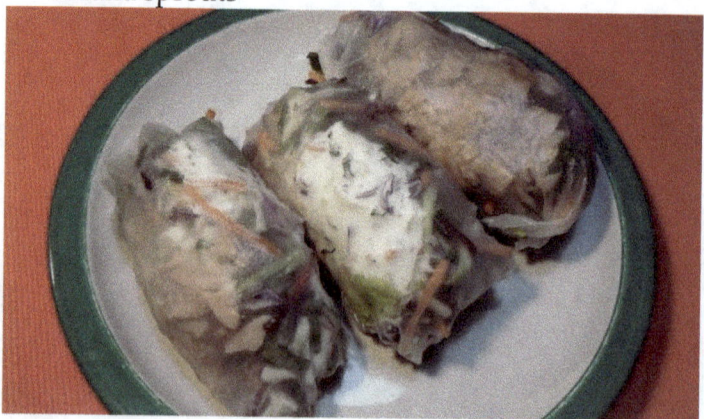

66. Tuna, balsamic, dill, alfalfa

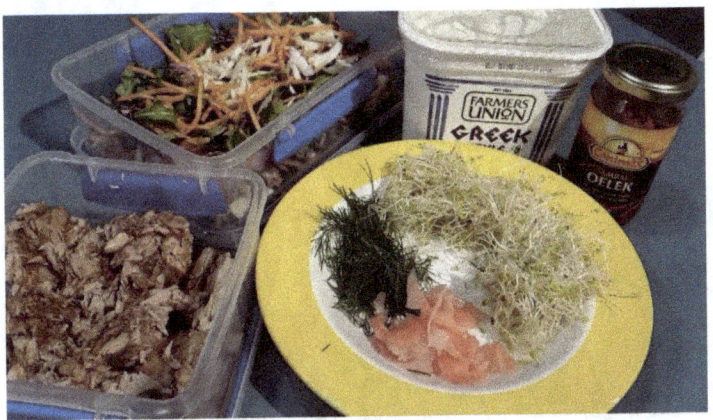

- 3 rice paper rounds
- 150g tinned tuna in springwater, drained
- Balsamic vinegar
- Greek yoghurt
- Conimex Sambal Oelek
- Pandaroo Sushi Ginger
- Mixed Crunchy Coleslaw Salad/Thai Mizuna Salad kit
- Alfalfa sprouts
- Fresh dill

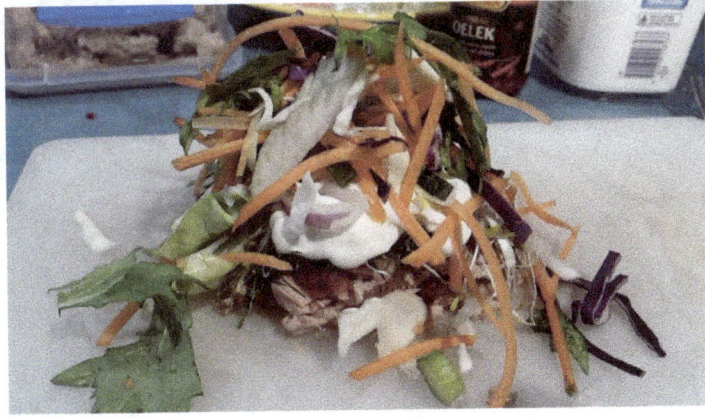

67. Tuna, balsamic, mizuna, dill

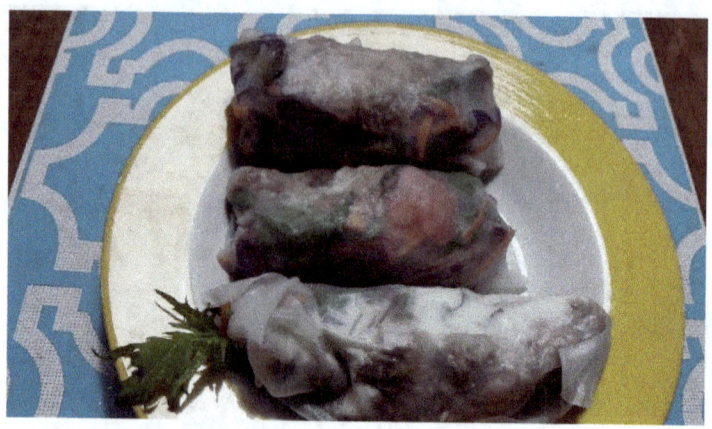

- 3 rice paper rounds
- 150g tinned tuna in springwater, drained
- Balsamic vinegar
- Greek yoghurt
- Pandaroo Sushi Ginger
- Pickled jalapenos, sliced
- Thai mizuna salad kit
- Fresh dill

68. Tuna, balsamic, mizuna, onion flakes

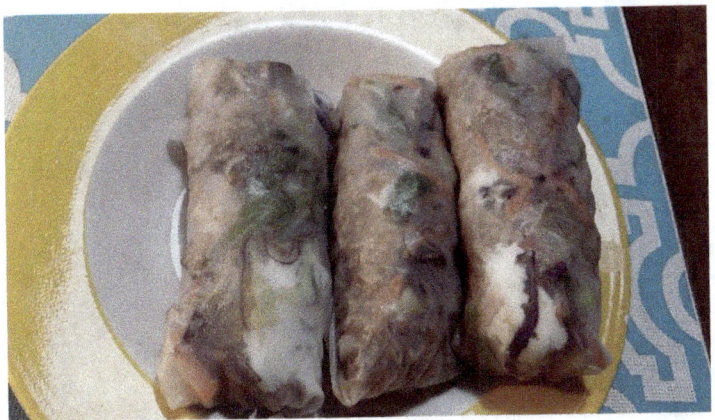

- 3 rice paper rounds
- 150g tinned tuna in springwater, drained
- Balsamic vinegar
- Greek yoghurt
- Pickled jalapenos, sliced
- Coleslaw
- Thai mizuna salad kit
- ½ packet of Crispy Onion Flakes from the salad pack

69. Tuna, balsamic, onion, lime

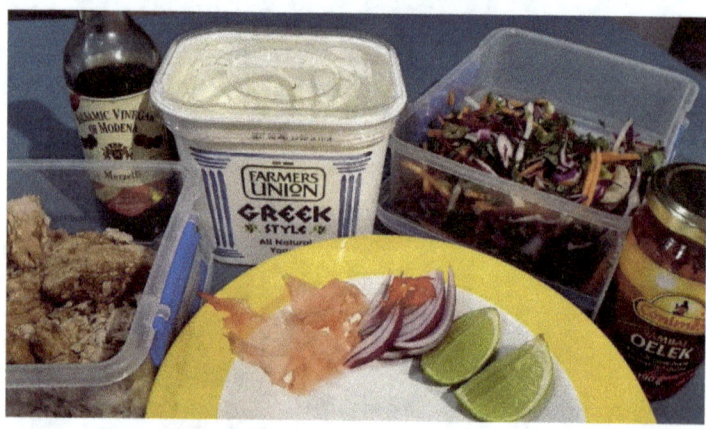

- 3 rice paper rounds
- 150g tinned tuna in springwater, drained
- Balsamic vinegar
- Greek yoghurt
- Conimex Sambal Oelek
- Pandaroo Sushi Ginger
- Fresh red onion and red chilli, thinly sliced
- Kaleslaw
- Lime juice

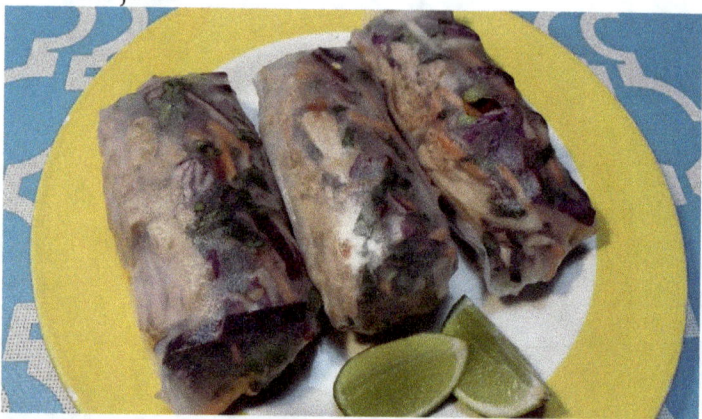

70. Tuna, balsamic, dill, tartare sauce

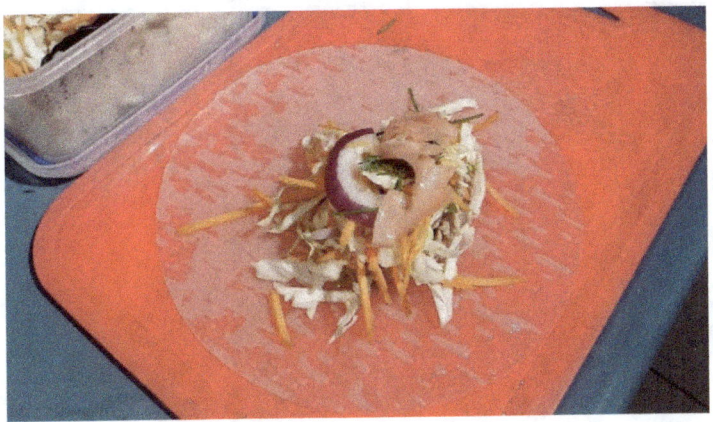

- 3 rice paper rounds
- 150g tinned tuna in springwater, drained
- Balsamic vinegar
- Pandaroo Sushi Ginger
- Coleslaw with onion
- Tartare sauce
- Fresh dill

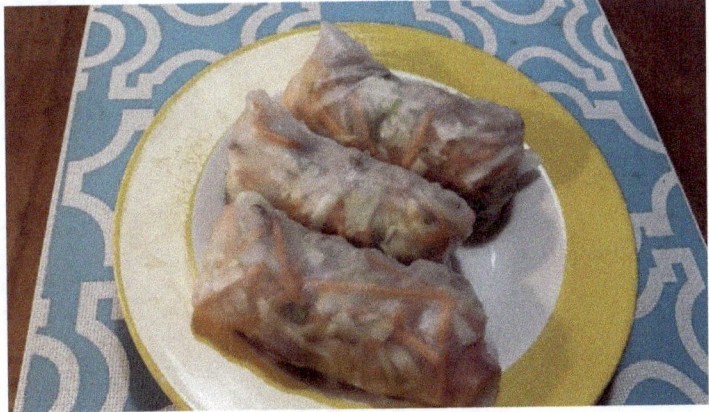

71. Tuna, balsamic, coleslaw, alfalfa

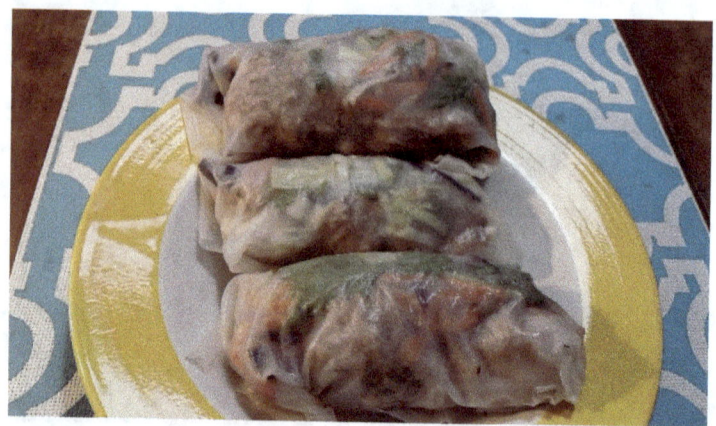

- 3 rice paper rounds
- 150g tinned tuna in springwater, drained
- Balsamic vinegar
- Pandaroo Sushi Ginger
- Coleslaw with dressing
- Alfalfa sprouts

72. Tuna, balsamic, Gochujang, lettuce

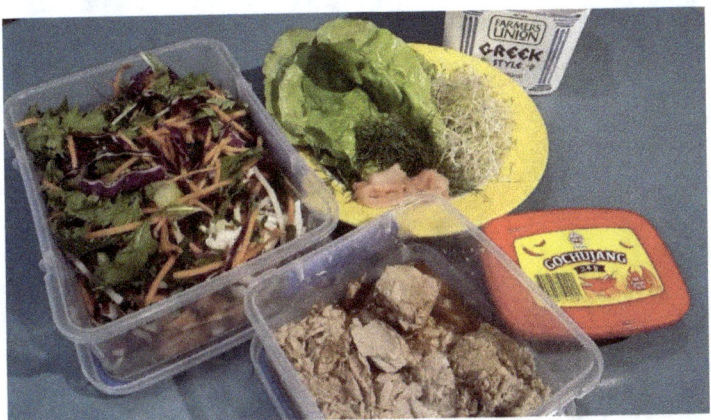

- 3 rice paper rounds
- 150g tinned tuna in springwater, drained
- Balsamic vinegar
- Gochujang chilli paste (very mild chilli)
- Pandaroo Sushi Ginger
- Mixed Crunchy Coleslaw/Kaleslaw/Thai Mizuna salad
- Butter lettuce
- Alfalfa sprouts
- Fresh dill

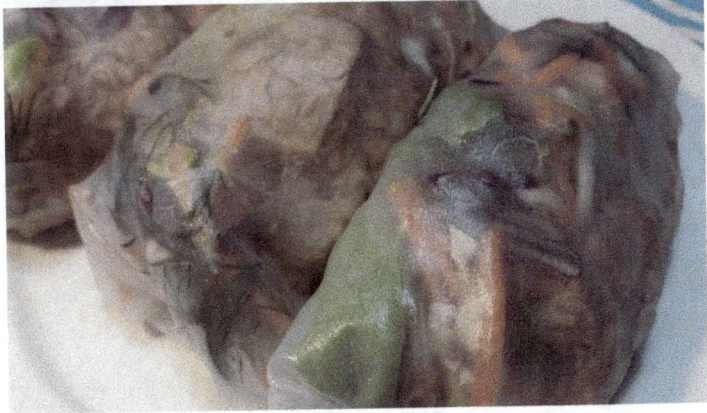

73. Tuna, kalamata, chilli, basil

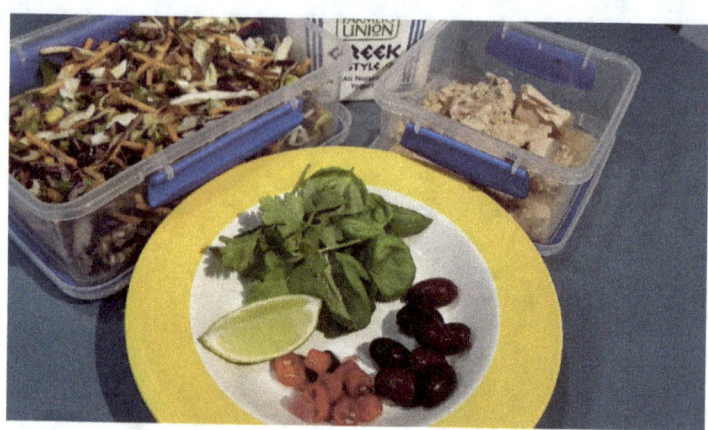

- 3 rice paper rounds
- 150g tinned tuna in springwater, drained
- Greek yoghurt
- Pickled red chilli
- Black olives
- Mixed coleslaw with dressing
- Fresh herbs (basil, parsley)

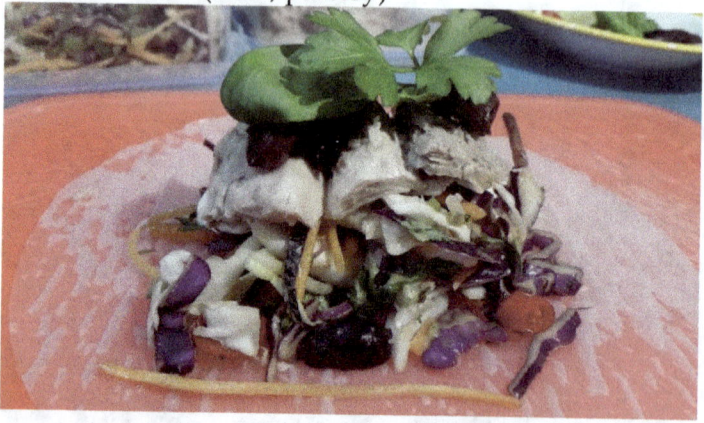

74. Tuna, tomato, mizuna, tartare sauce

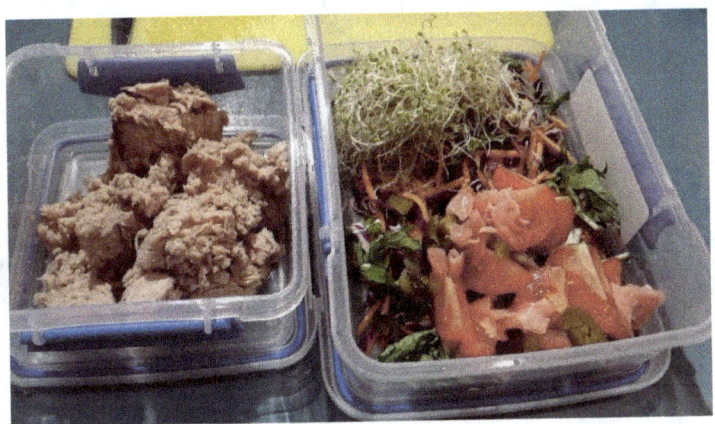

- 3 rice paper rounds
- 150g tinned tuna in springwater, drained
- Pandaroo Sushi Ginger
- 1 small tomato, chopped
- Tartare sauce
- Thai mizuna salad kit
- Alfalfa sprouts

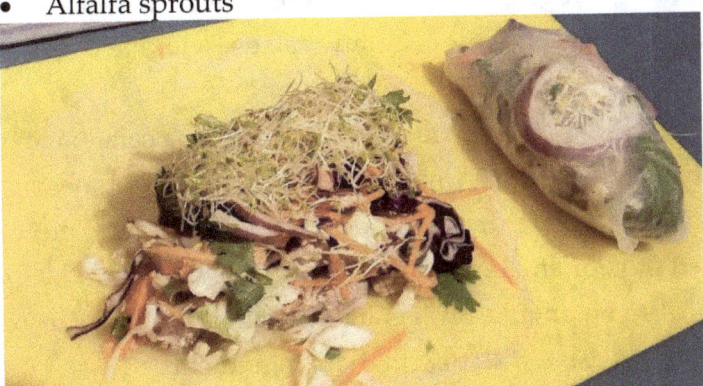

TUNA SALAD BOWLS

Who doesn't love a salad bowl? And these tuna salads will satisfy the mouth and the belly. Fresh, flavourful, and filling, these salads will make you smile. But be careful. Don't be heavy-handed with the portions. Use a small bowl and eat slowly.

Salads are simple to make for lunch or dinner. They are easily transported to the office, the beach, or a friend's place for a casual get-together. No need to feel concerned about your food choices, as these yummy salads will have everyone envious.

The simplest way to approach making a salad is to open the fridge door to see what you have on hand. You need some salad vegetables, a dressing, and some extra bits and pieces for added flavour and texture.

As you should always have the makings for rice paper rolls, I suggest you start with those ingredients:
- Some type of coleslaw, kaleslaw, or other salad veges
- 200g tinned tuna in springwater, drained
- A few slices of Sushi Ginger
- A few slices of pickled jalapenos
- ½ fresh ripe tomato, chopped or sliced
- A dollop of Greek yoghurt
- Some Asian herbs

- And a dressing, such as a Poonsin Vietnamese dipping sauce, or a vinaigrette of lime juice and sesame oil.
- To make your mouth happy, top with something crunchy or extra tasty (like crushed nuts, fried onion flakes, or pineapple).

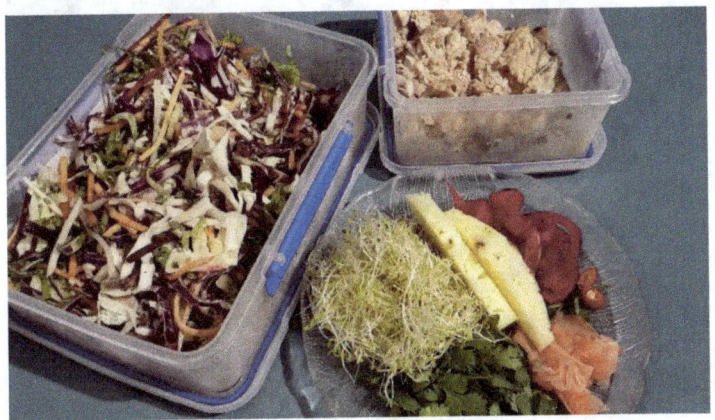

If not using rice papers or rice noodles, you can increase the protein to 200g of tuna.

If not using yoghurt, you can increase the avocado from ¼ to ½ per meal, if desired.

75. Tuna, mizuna salad, onion flakes

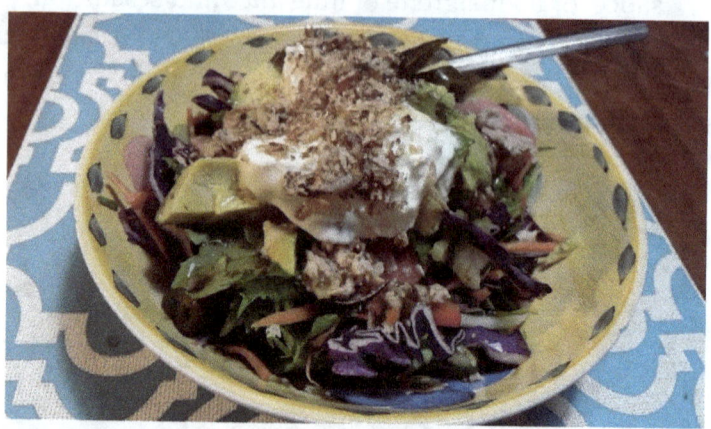

- 200g tinned tuna in springwater, drained
- Dollop of Greek yoghurt
- ½ avocado
- Pandaroo Sushi Ginger
- Pickled jalapenos, sliced
- Thai mizuna salad kit
- Kaleslaw
- Sprinkle with ½ packet of fried onion pieces from Thai mizuna Salad kit

76. Spicy tuna, tomato, dill salad

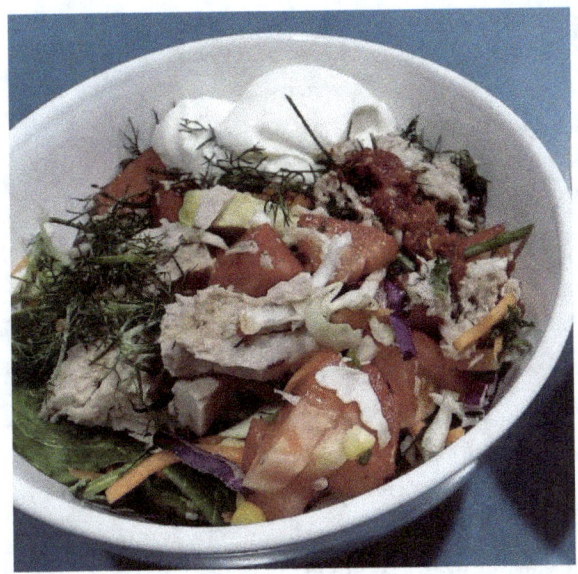

- 200g tinned tuna in springwater, drained
- Dollop of Greek yoghurt
- ¼ avocado
- 1 x tomato, sliced
- Conimex Sambal Oelek
- Mixed coleslaw
- Fresh herbs (dill, fennel)

77. Spicy tuna, yoghurt salad

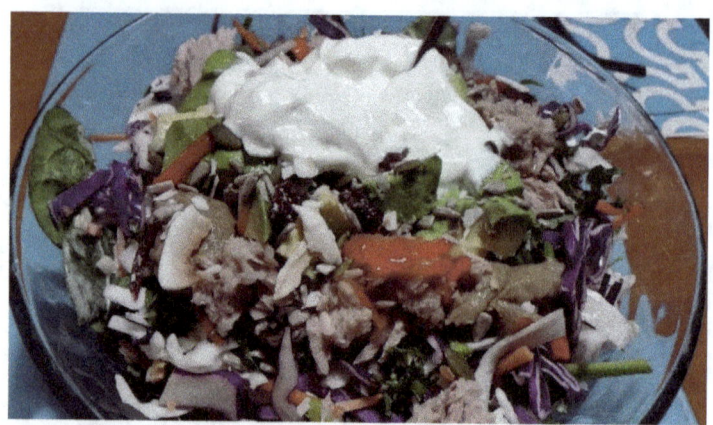

- 200g tinned tuna, drained
- Dollop of Greek yoghurt
- ¼ avocado, sliced
- Pickled jalapenos, sliced
- Conimex Sambal Oelek
- Tablespoon of tahini paste
- Splash of Poonsin Vietnamese Spring Roll Dipping Sauce
- Mixed baby lettuce leaves
- Mixed coleslaw
- Sprinkle with packet of mixed seeds from salad pack

78. Tuna, pineapple, crunchy noodle salad

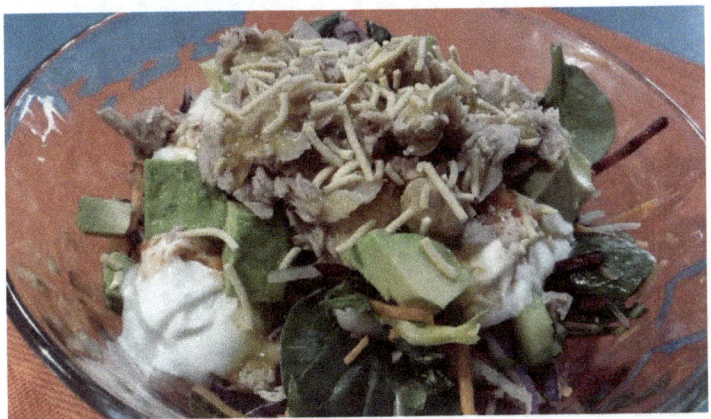

- 200g tinned tuna in springwater, drained
- Greek yoghurt
- ¼ avocado
- Slice of tinned pineapple, chopped
- Conimex Sambal Oelek
- Mixed coleslaw
- Splash of Poonsin Vietnamese Spring Roll Dipping Sauce
- Sprinkle with ½ packet of crunchy fried noodles from coleslaw kit

79. Tuna and warm asparagus salad

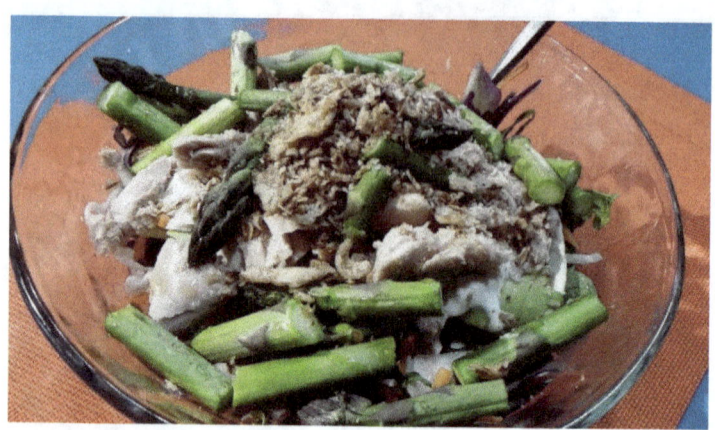

In a heated frypan,
- add a teaspoon of sesame oil
- add a bunch of asparagus, chopped
- quickly stir-fry for a couple of minutes, then take off the heat

In a serving bowl, construct your salad:
- mixed coleslaw and baby lettuce leaves
- Greek yoghurt
- ¼ avocado
- Fresh red chilli, chopped
- 200g tinned tuna in springwater, drained
- Tablespoon of tahini paste
- Cooked asparagus from frypan
- Sprinkle with ½ packet of dried onion flakes from Thai mizuna salad kit

80. Tuna, Caesar rainbow salad

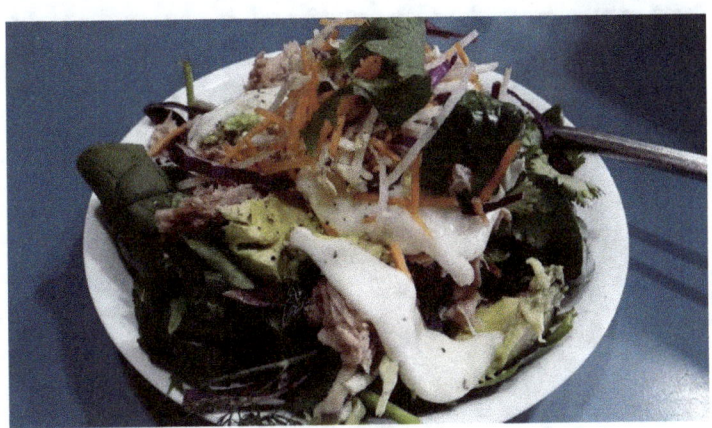

- 200g tinned tuna in springwater, drained
- ½ avocado
- Pickled jalapenos, sliced
- Caesar salad dressing
- Baby spinach and other leaves
- Rainbow coleslaw (shredded vegetables)

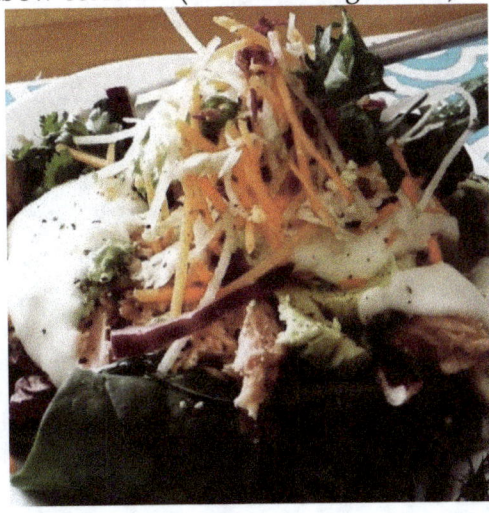

81. Italian tuna, balsamic, olive salad

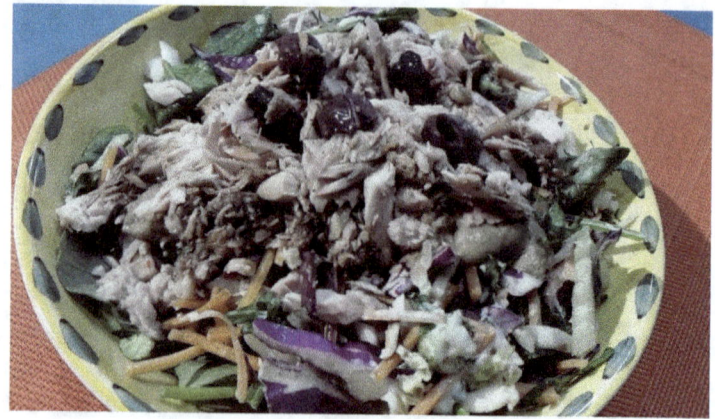

- 200g tinned tuna, drained
- ½ avocado, sliced
- Splash of Balsamic vinegar
- ½ cup black Kalamata olives, seeds removed
- Tablespoon of tahini paste
- Mixed baby lettuce leaves with shredded carrot
- Mixed coleslaw, with dressing

82. Italian tuna, olive, tomato salad

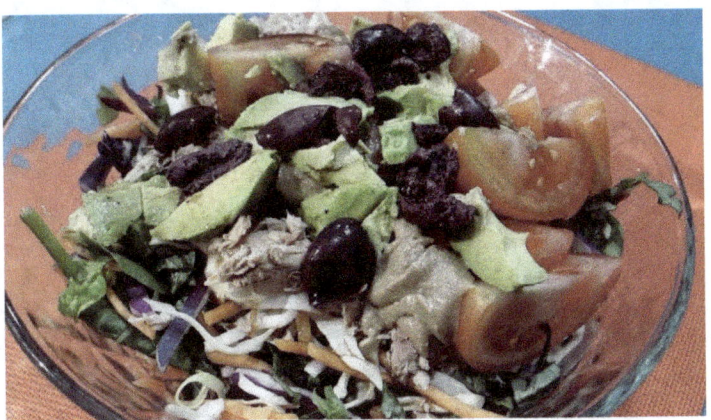

- 200g tinned tuna, drained
- ½ avocado, sliced
- Splash of Balsamic vinegar
- ½ cup black Kalamata olives, seeds removed
- 1 x ripe tomato, cut into chunks
- Tablespoon of tahini paste
- Mixed baby lettuce leaves
- Mixed coleslaw/kaleslaw, with dressing
- Season to taste

83. Spicy Italian tuna, basil salad

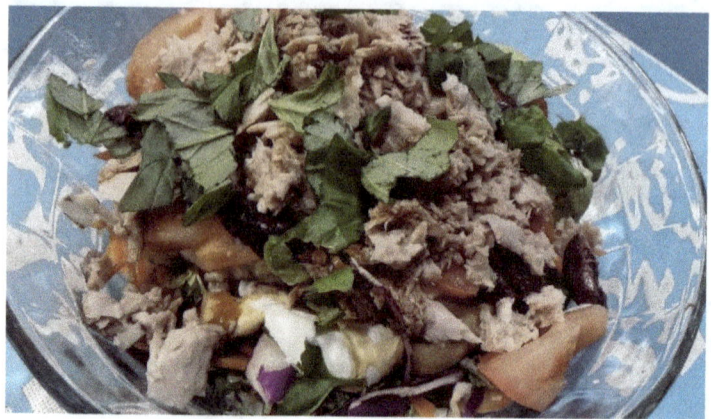

- 200g tinned tuna, drained
- Greek yoghurt
- ¼ avocado, sliced
- Balsamic vinegar
- ½ cup black Kalamata olives, seeds removed
- 1 x ripe tomato, cut into chunks
- Tablespoon of tahini paste
- Conimex Sambal Oelek
- Mixed baby lettuce leaves
- Mixed coleslaw
- Fresh basil

84. Italian tuna, tomato, artichoke salad

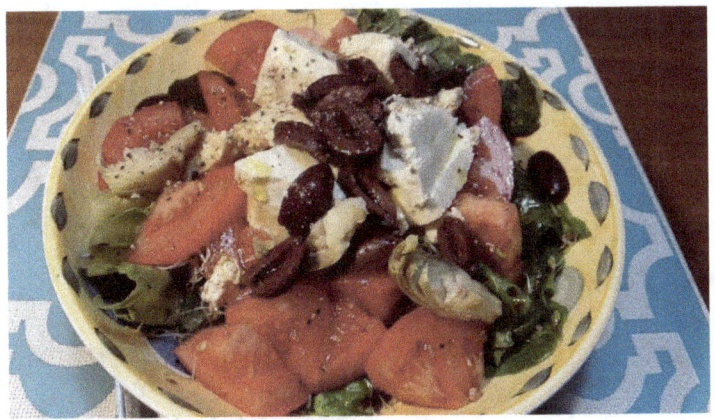

- 200g tinned tuna, drained
- 2 x pickled artichokes, in quarters
- Vinaigrette dressing
    - Splash of Balsamic vinegar
    - Splash of extra virgin olive oil
    - A few drops of sesame oil
- ½ cup black Kalamata olives, seeds removed
- 1 x large ripe tomato, cut into chunks
- Mixed baby lettuce leaves
- Mixed coleslaw
- Fresh basil

85. The Traveller, tuna, noodle salad

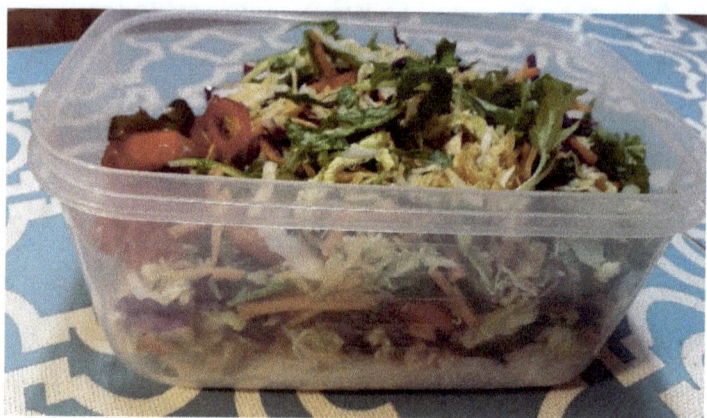

- Single serve of reconstituted rice vermicelli noodles, chilled
- 150g tinned tuna in springwater, drained
- ½ fresh tomato, chopped
- Jalapenos
- Chili
- Poonsin Vietnamese spring roll dipping sauce

To keep salad crisp while transporting, add wet ingredients first, then top with dry salad veges:
- Mixed Asian coleslaw/Thai mizuna salad kit
- Onion flakes

86. Tuna, coleslaw, noodle salad

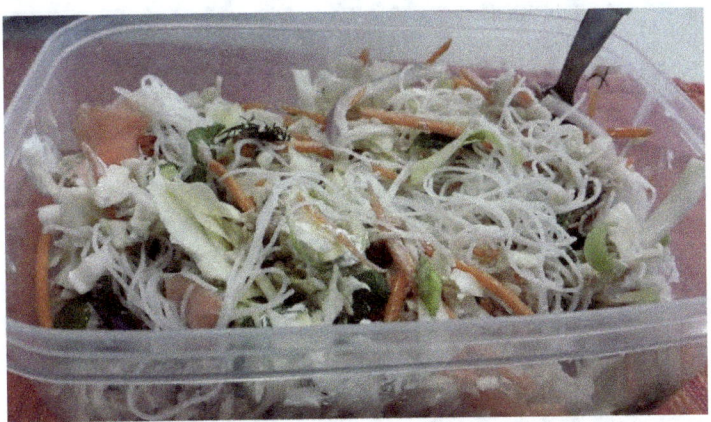

- Vermicelli noodles, reconstituted and chilled
- 150g tinned tuna in springwater, drained
- Greek yoghurt
- ¼ avocado
- Pandaroo Sushi Ginger
- Fresh red chilli, chopped
- Crunchy Coleslaw with onion rings
- Grated fennel bulb
- Fresh dill

87. Tonkatsu tuna with warm noodle salad

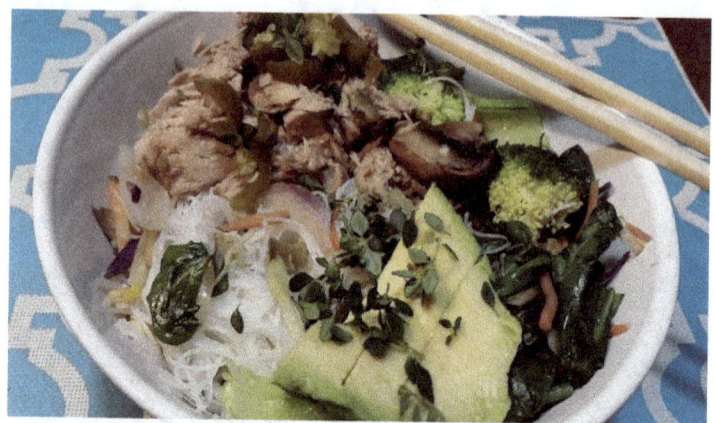

Stir-fry veges in hot pan with olive oil and sesame oil (broccoli, mushrooms, bok choy, Rainbow Stir-fry veg)

Serve in a bowl with:

- ½ serve vermicelli noodles
- ¼ avocado
- Cold 150g tinned tuna in springwater, drained with balsamic vinegar
- Pickled jalapenos, sliced
- Fresh lemon thyme
- Japanese Obentu brand Tonkatsu Sauce

TINNED TUNA in SOUPS

With just a few basic ingredients, you can create spicy curries, tomato-based stews, and simple broths. But avoid adding too many competing flavours and textures, or the result can taste muddy and bland. So, keep it simple, and keep it fresh.

The recipes in this section appear in 'HOW TO COOK FISH', the first cookbook in this series, but you can use them for tinned fish too. They are a quick and easy way of USING LEFTOVERS – especially salad vegetables, lettuce, and the last dregs of tuna in that plastic container in the fridge.

Seriously though, you can toss almost anything into a frypan and make it delicious, especially in wintertime. And by adding a portion of cheap protein – tuna, pink salmon, or even tofu – you have a tasty meal which is good for your belly and your pocket.

Anyone can make these dishes. You don't have to know how to cook! Just add heat and throw it all in. No finesse required. Great use of leftover bits and pieces you have in the fridge.

88. Indian yellow curry noodle soup

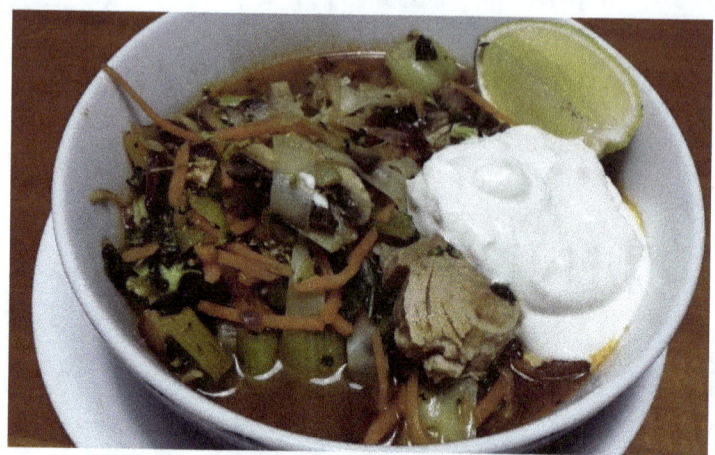

- Prepare a serve of flat rice noodles by cooking in a saucepan of boiling water for a few minutes. Drain and set aside.

To a hot pan, add a splash of olive oil, sliced mushrooms, salt, cracked pepper. Allow mushrooms to fry for a few minutes.

- Add chopped broccoli, Asian leafy greens (gai lan or choy sum)
- Add cup of mixed coleslaw salad vegetables
- Mix large teaspoon of Yellow Curry Paste (Indian style) with a cup of water. Add to pan and bring to boil.
- Add 200g tinned tuna, in chunks
- Cover with lid and simmer for a few minutes.
- Serve in a bowl with flat rice noodles
- Top with a squeeze of lime juice and dollop of yoghurt.

89. Malaysian Laksa noodle soup

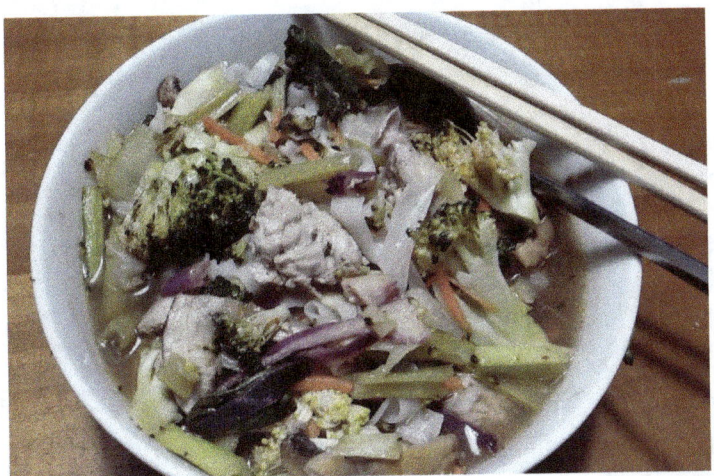

- Prepare a serve of flat rice noodles by cooking in a saucepan of boiling water for a few minutes. Drain and set aside.

To a hot pan, add a splash of olive oil, sliced mushrooms, salt, cracked pepper. Allow to fry for a few minutes.

- Add chopped broccoli, Asian leafy greens (gai lan or choy sum)
- Add cup of mixed coleslaw salad vegetables
- Mix large teaspoon of Malaysian Laksa Paste with a cup of water. Add to pan and bring to boil.
- Add 200g tinned tuna, in chunks
- Add splash of fish sauce, and vinegar
- Serve in a bowl with flat rice noodles
- Add lime juice and dollop of yoghurt, if desired.

90. Instant Vietnamese pho

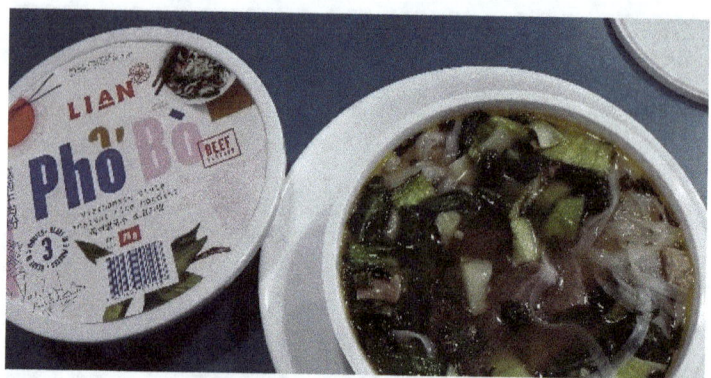

Lian Pho Bo Vietnamese Style instant rice noodle soup, 70g, with flavour sachets, in a plastic bowl

- Open the flavour sachets and sprinkle them over the dried vermicelli noodles in the plastic bowl. Then cover with boiling water until about an inch from the rim.
- Loosely cover with lid for a couple of minutes.
- Remove lid and stir softened noodles.
- Add baby bok choy, chopped
- Add 200g tinned tuna
- Cover with lid for a couple of minutes until the bok choy is wilted
- Serve with a side plate of Vietnamese-style toppings (coriander, Vietnamese mint, lemon juice, chili).
- If required, balance flavours with a dash of soy and/or fish sauce.

91. Thai Tom Yum vege soup

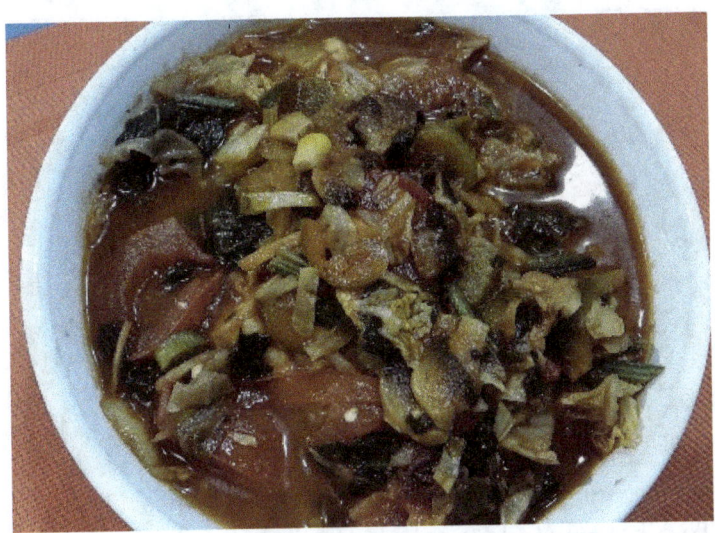

To a hot pan, add olive oil, teaspoon Tom Yum Paste, habanero mild chili, salt, cracked pepper
- Add sliced mushrooms. Fry until browned.
- Add vegetables (spinach, coleslaw, shredded wombok)
- Add 200g of tinned fish
- Mix ½ cup tomato passata, ½ tin tomato pieces, ½ cup water. Pour over fish.
- Stir in a teaspoon of tamarind puree to balance flavours
- Cover with lid. Simmer for a couple of minutes until the veges soften and the tomato flavours get a chance to mellow.
- Serve with fresh lime juice

92. Thai Tom Yum noodle braise

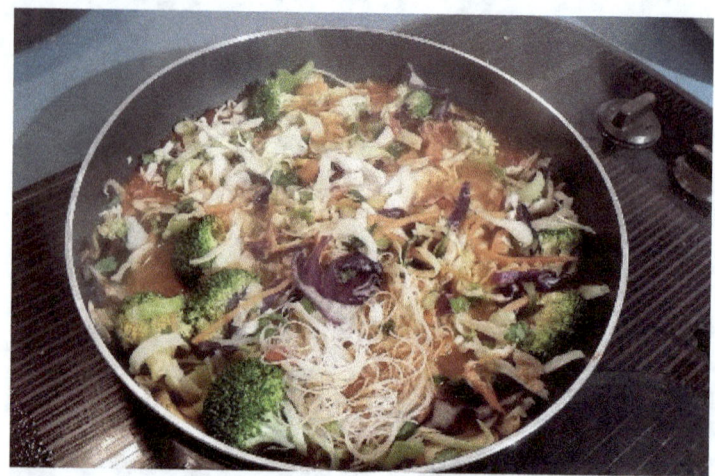

- Reconstitute a serve of vermicelli noodles. Drain.

To a hot pan, add a splash of olive oil, sliced mushrooms, chopped shallots, salt, cracked pepper. Allow to fry for a few minutes.

- Add sliced broccoli (or ½ cup frozen peas)
- Add a cup of mixed coleslaw veg
- Stir in a teaspoon of Tom Yum paste and a teaspoon of Tamarind Puree
- Add 200g tinned tina
- Mix ½ cup tomato passata, ½ tin tomato pieces, ½ cup water. Pour over fish.
- Add drained noodles. Cover with lid. Allow to cook for a couple of minutes.
- Serve in a bowl with fresh lime juice

93. Hoisin, broccoli, noodle braise

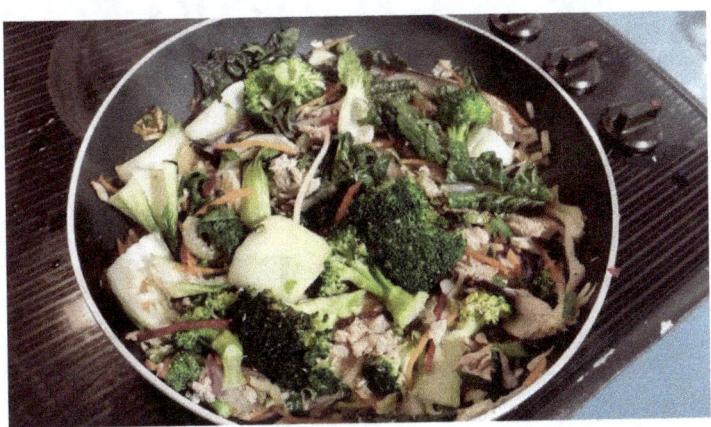

- In a bowl, pour boiling water over dried vermicelli noodles

To a hot pan, add olive oil, teaspoon of sambal oelek, teaspoon Hoisin sauce

- Add chopped greens (silverbeet, bok choy, broccoli)
- Add cup of mixed salad veg (coleslaw/kaleslaw)
- Add 200g tinned tuna, drained
- Add a cup of stock
- Add cooked vermicelli noodles, drained
- Cover with lid. Simmer until broccoli stems have softened.
- Serve with Viet mint, Thai basil, and a splash of fish sauce. Lemon juice is optional.

TINNED PINK SALMON

In Asian-style salad recipes, I prefer the taste and texture of tinned tuna over tinned pink salmon. But if you choose to use pink salmon, be aware of the differences:

- Salmon contains more of the omega-3 fats than tuna, but this is why salmon also has more calories per 100g.
- Tinned salmon is always packed in brine (salty water), so if you buy tuna packed in SPRINGWATER, you ingest less salt. This is an important consideration for many people.
- Some brands of tinned pink salmon can smell and taste a bit too fishy for my liking, especially the cheaper brands. Pink salmon can benefit from being mashed with a splash of vinegar and/or the addition of chopped onion, especially for salads. The mashed bones provide dietary calcium.
- Pink salmon comes into its own when used in cooked dishes where the strong flavour is beneficial.

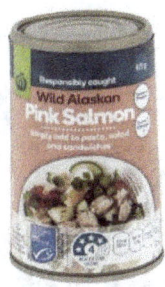

While pink salmon is not my favourtie, I have tried many different brands from major supermarkets. I keep coming back to **WOOLWORTHS'** Wild Alaskan PINK Salmon (415g) for taste, texture, and price.

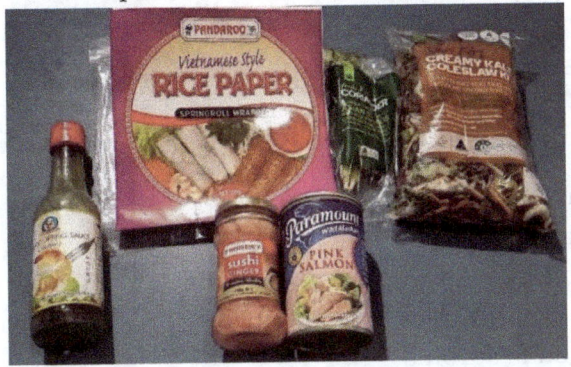

PARAMOUNT Wild Alaskan PINK Salmon (415g) is an economical choice too, but it's best if you discard the skin before mashing.

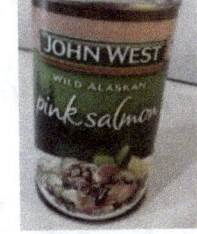

JOHN WEST Wild Alaskan PINK Salmon (415g), as one would expect, has excellent taste and texture, but at a much higher price point.

94. Pink salmon, creamy avo, chilli

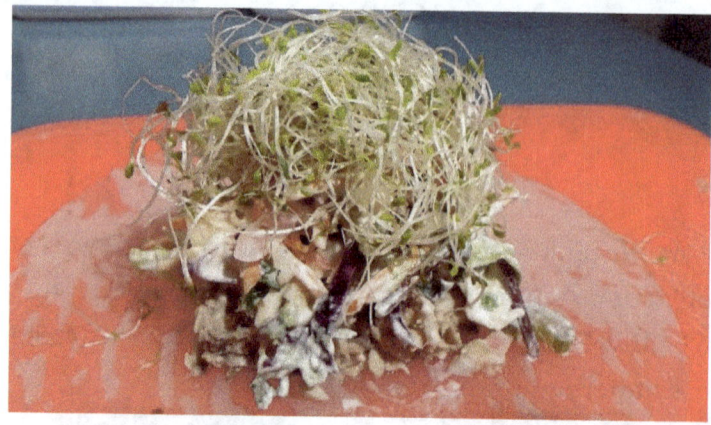

- 3 rice paper rounds
- 150g Woolworth's PINK salmon, drained
- Greek yoghurt
- ½ avocado
- Fresh red chilli, chopped
- Pandaroo Sushi Ginger
- Southern style coleslaw kit with dressing
- Kaleslaw
- Alfalfa sprouts

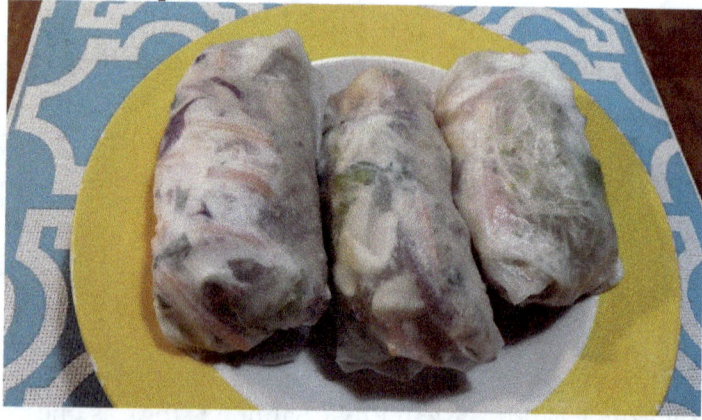

95. Pink salmon, spicy southern dressing

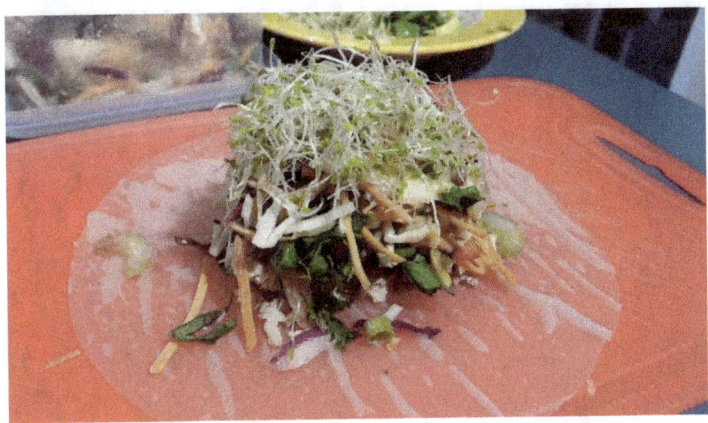

- 3 rice paper rounds
- 150g Woolworth's PINK salmon, drained
- ½ avocado
- Fresh red chilli, chopped
- Lime juice
- Southern style coleslaw kit with dressing
- Alfalfa sprouts

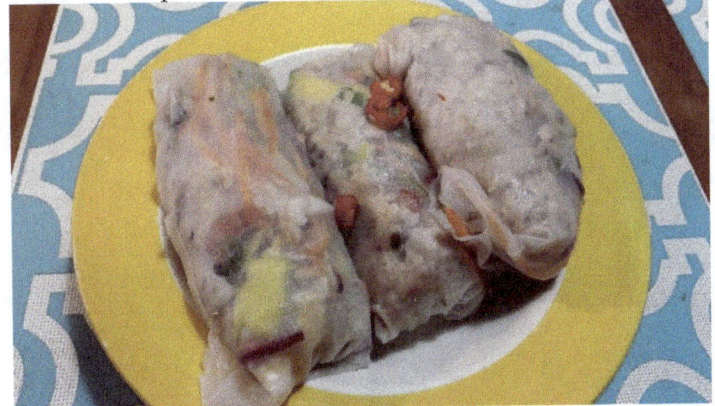

96. Pink salmon, sauerkraut, gherkin

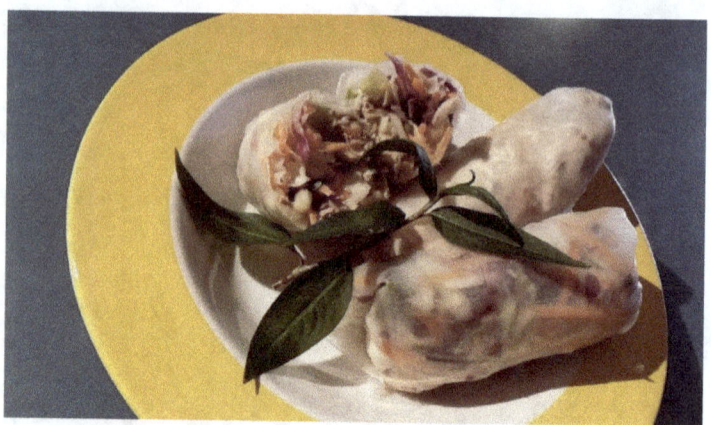

- 3 rice paper rounds
- 150g Woolworth's PINK salmon, drained
- Greek yoghurt
- Sauerkraut
- Pickled gherkin, chopped
- Conimex Sambal Oelek
- Coleslaw, dry
- Alfalfa sprouts
- Fresh Vietnamese mint

97. Pink salmon, pineapple, capsicum

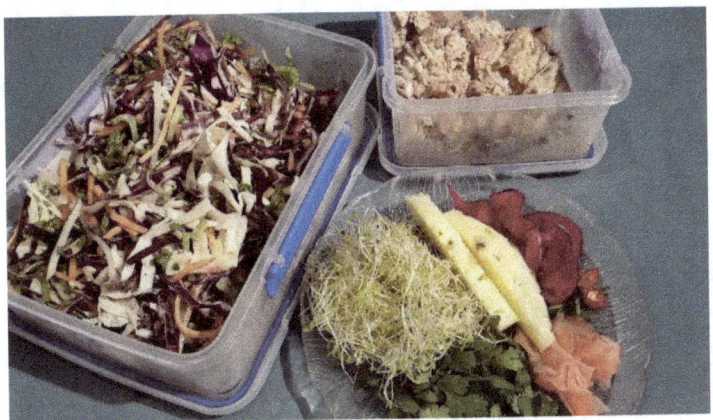

- 3 rice paper rounds
- 150g Woolworth's PINK salmon, drained
- Pandaroo Sushi Ginger
- Fresh pineapple, sliced
- Fresh red capsicum, sliced
- Pickled onion with chilli, chopped
- Mix coleslaw/kaleslaw with dressing
- Alfalfa sprouts
- Fresh coriander

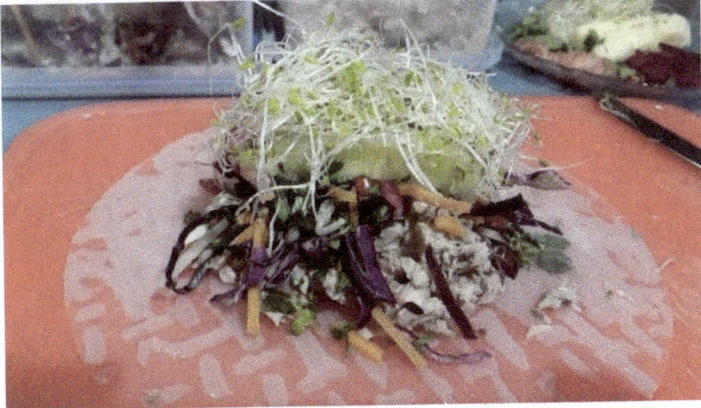

98. Pink salmon, mild chilli, lime

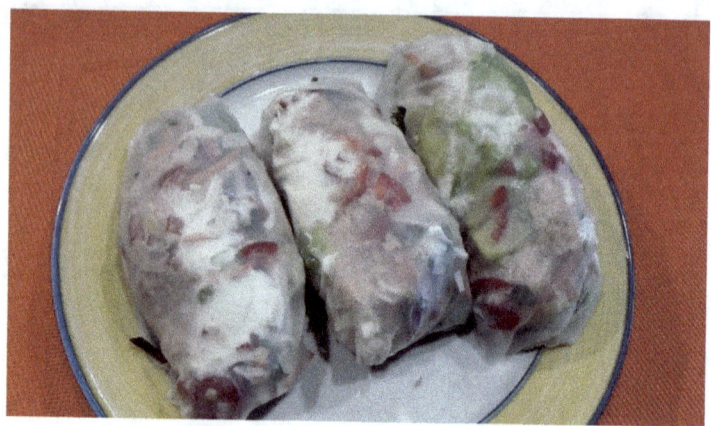

- 3 rice paper rounds
- 150g Woolworth's PINK salmon, drained
- Greek yoghurt
- ¼ avocado
- Fresh mild habanero chilli, chopped
- Mixed coleslaw/kaleslaw
- Mixed lettuce leaves
- Lime juice

99. Pink salmon, dill, nori

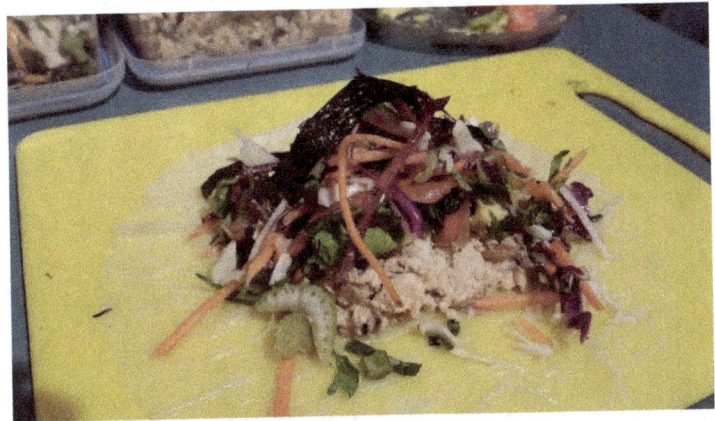

- 3 rice paper rounds
- 150g Woolworth's PINK salmon, drained
- ½ avocado
- Pandaroo Sushi Ginger
- Pickled jalapenos, chopped
- Pickled red chilli, chopped
- Southern Style Coleslaw/kaleslaw, with dressing
- Fresh dill
- Nori strips

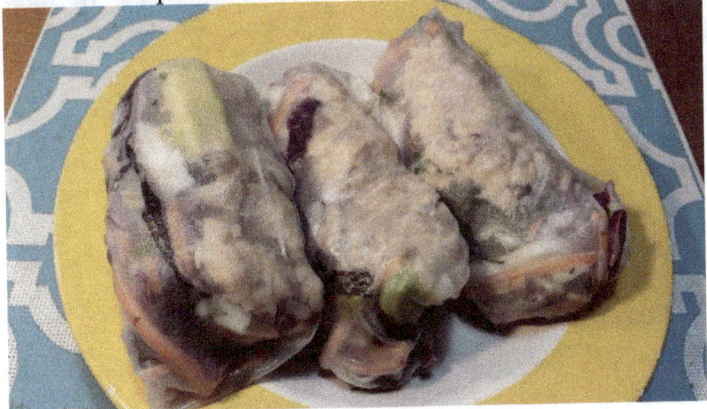

100. Pink salmon, dill, Viet sauce

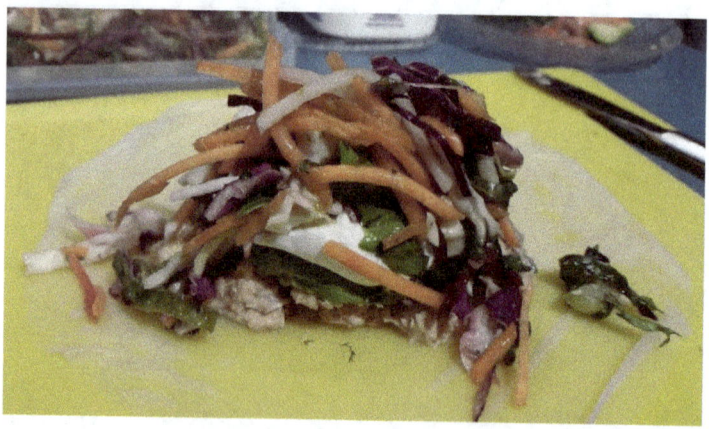

- 3 rice paper rounds
- 150g Woolworth's PINK salmon, drained
- Greek yoghurt
- ¼ avocado
- Pandaroo Sushi Ginger
- Southern Style Coleslaw/kaleslaw, with dressing
- Fresh dill
- Poonsin Vietnamese Spring Roll Dipping Sauce

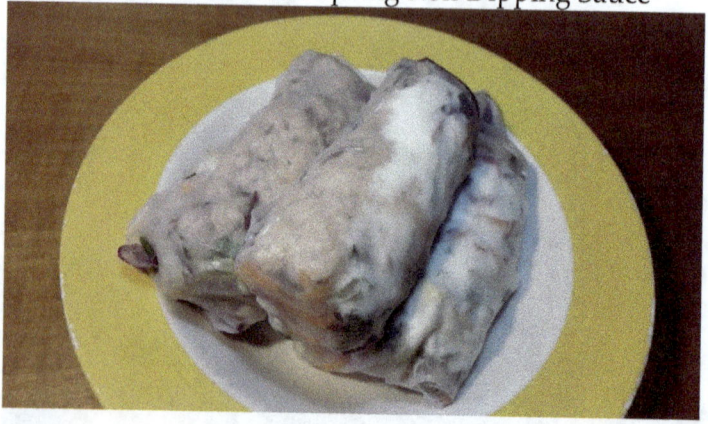

101. Pink salmon, pickled ginger juice

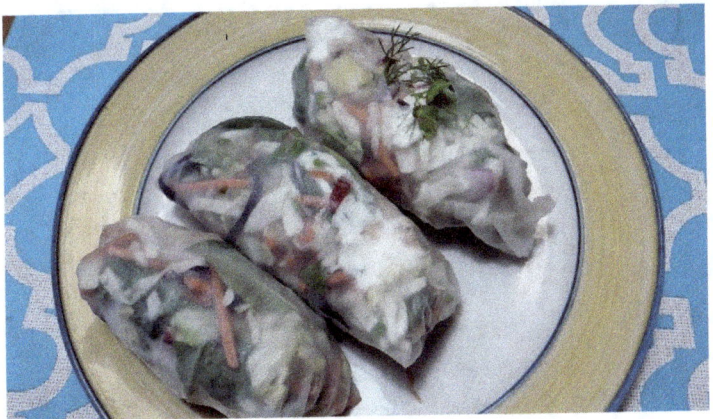

- 3 rice paper rounds
- 150g Woolworth's PINK salmon, drained
- Greek yoghurt
- ¼ avocado
- Pandaroo Sushi Ginger
- Fresh red chilli, chopped
- Mixed coleslaw
- Drizzle of sweet tangy juice from Sushi Ginger bottle

102. Pink salmon, prawns, herbs, lime

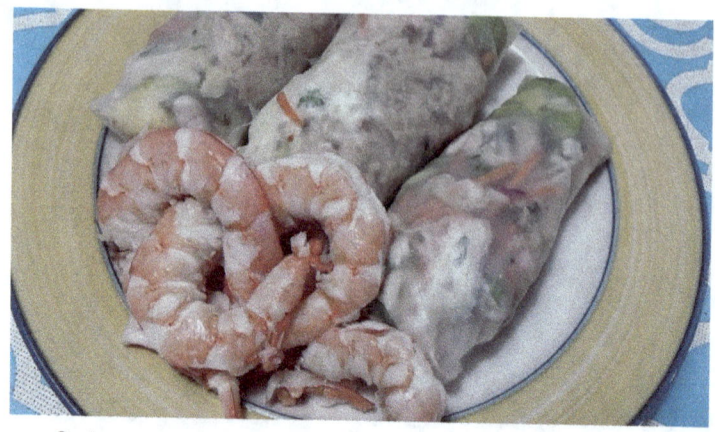

- 3 rice paper rounds
- 150g Woolworth's PINK salmon, drained
- Greek yoghurt
- ¼ avocado
- Pandaroo Sushi Ginger
- Fresh red chilli, chopped
- Mixed coleslaw
- Fresh Asian herbs
- Serve with 4 peeled prawns on the side, and lime juice

103. Pink salmon, prawns, pineapple, mint

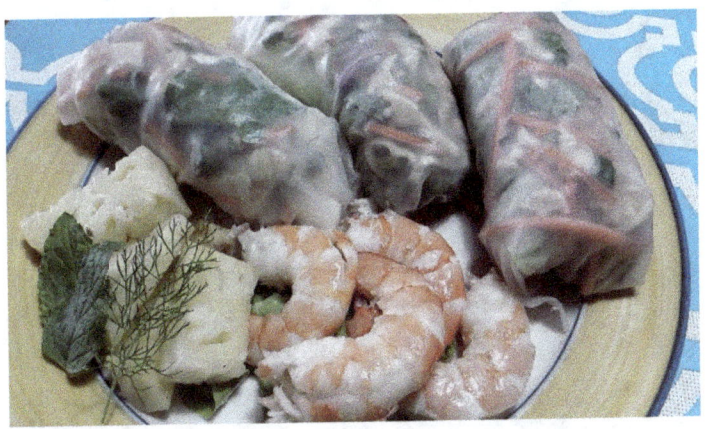

- 3 rice paper rounds
- 150g Woolworth's PINK salmon, drained
- Greek yoghurt
- Fresh red chilli, chopped
- Mixed kaleslaw/coleslaw
- Lettuce
- Fresh herbs (garden mint, fennel)
- Serve with
    - 4 peeled prawns on the side
    - Fresh pineapple, sliced
    - Fresh garden mint
    - Fresh lime

104. Pink salmon, prawns, pineapple, ginger

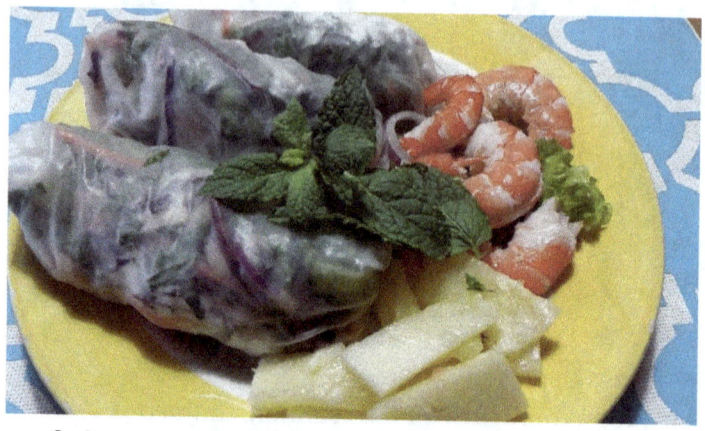

- 3 rice paper rounds
- 150g Woolworth's PINK salmon, drained
- Greek yoghurt
- Pandaroo Sushi Ginger
- Pickled jalapenos, chopped
- Mixed kaleslaw/coleslaw
- Serve with
    - 4 peeled prawns on the side
    - Fresh pineapple, sliced
    - Fresh garden mint

105. Pink salmon, chilli, Viet mint

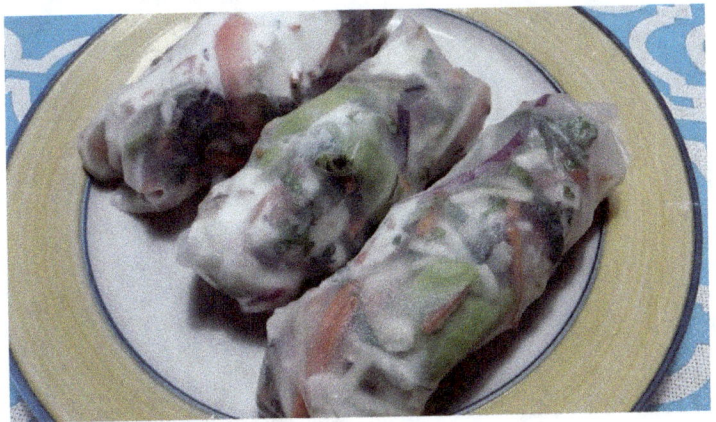

- 3 rice paper rounds
- 150g Woolworth's PINK salmon, drained
- Greek yoghurt
- ¼ avocado
- Pandaroo Sushi Ginger
- Fresh red chilli, chopped
- Mixed coleslaw/kaleslaw
- Fresh Vietnamese mint
- Lime juice

106. Pink salmon, coriander, Chang's

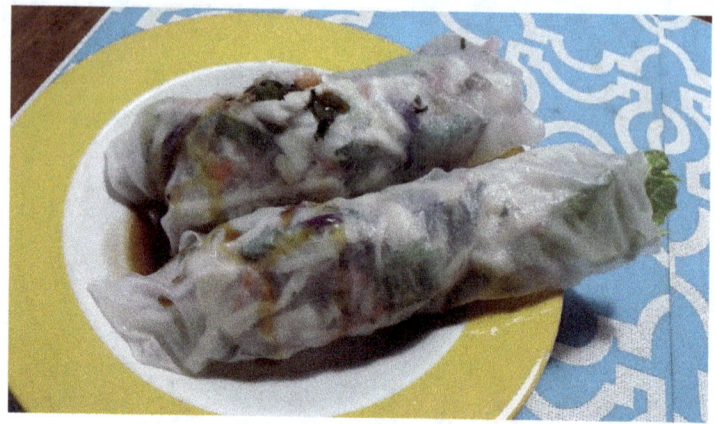

- 3 rice paper rounds
- 150g Paramount PINK salmon, drained
- Balsamic vinegar
- Mixed coleslaw
- Lettuce
- Fresh coriander
- Chang's Fried Noodle Dipping Sauce

107. Pink salmon, balsamic, coleslaw

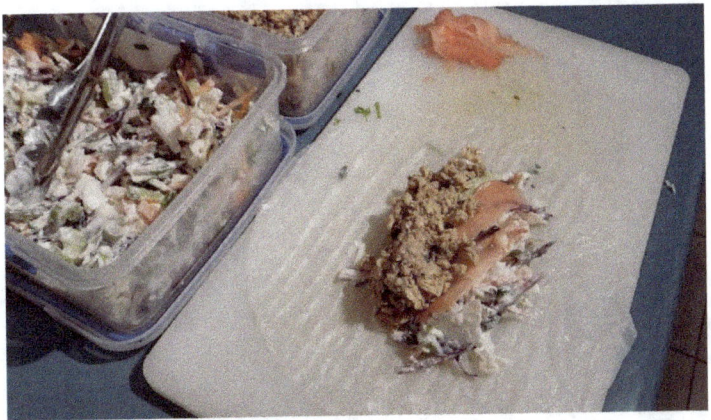

- 3 rice paper rounds
- 150g Paramount PINK salmon
- Balsamic vinegar
- Pandaroo Sushi Ginger
- Lazy mixed salad –
    - Dry coleslaw
    - Greek yoghurt
    - Pickled jalapenos, sliced
    - Fresh coriander
    - Poonsin Vietnamese spring roll dipping sauce

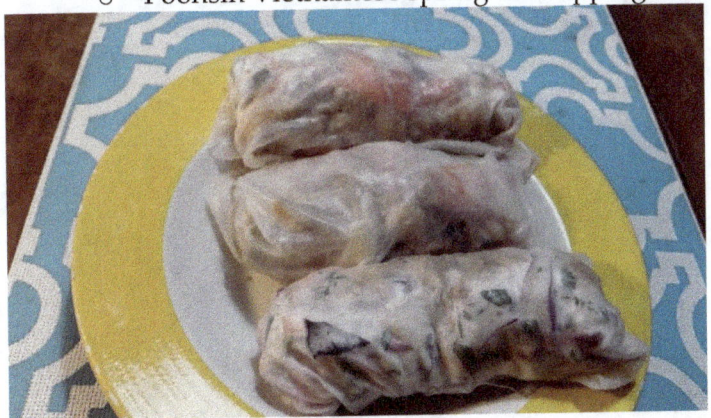

108. Pink salmon, tomato, mizuna

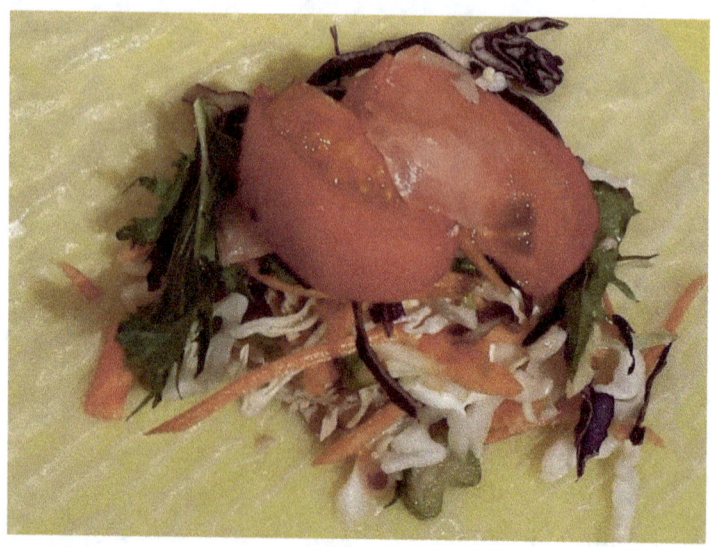

- 3 rice paper rounds
- 150g Paramount PINK salmon, drained
- Balsamic vinegar
- Greek yoghurt
- Pandaroo Sushi Ginger
- 1 x tomato, chopped
- Pickled jalapenos, chopped
- Mixed coleslaw / Thai mizuna salad kit

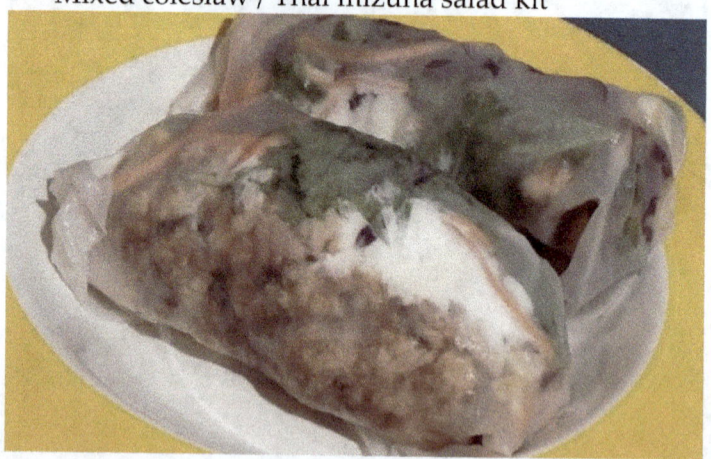

109. Pink salmon, nori, mizuna

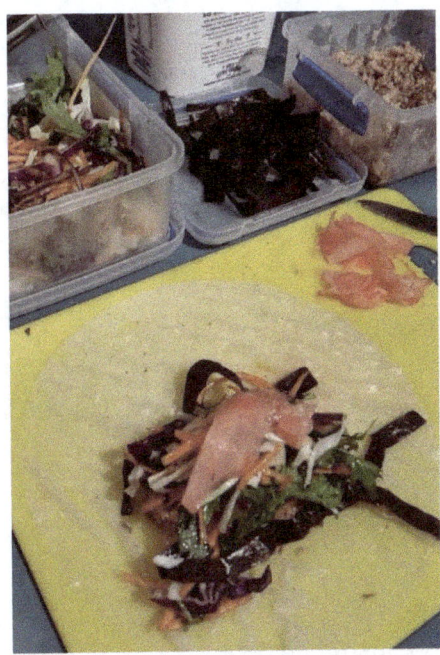

- 3 rice paper rounds
- 150g Paramount PINK salmon, drained
- Balsamic vinegar
- Greek yoghurt
- Pandaroo Sushi Ginger
- Fresh red chilli, chopped
- Mixed coleslaw
- Thai mizuna salad kit, with Thai dressing
- Nori strips

110. Pink salmon, chilli, Thai basil

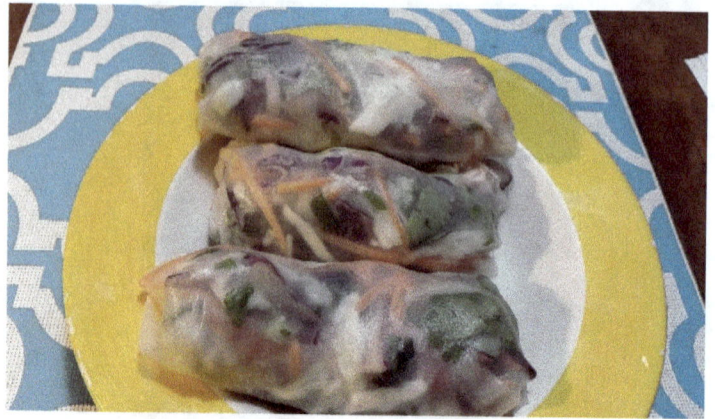

- 3 rice paper rounds
- 150g Paramount PINK salmon, drained
- Balsamic vinegar
- Greek yoghurt
- ½ avocado
- Pandaroo Sushi Ginger
- Pickled jalapenos, chopped
- Fresh red chilli, chopped
- Coleslaw veg, dry
- Kaleslaw, with dressing
- Fresh herbs (coriander, Thai basil)

111. Pink salmon, balsamic, coriander

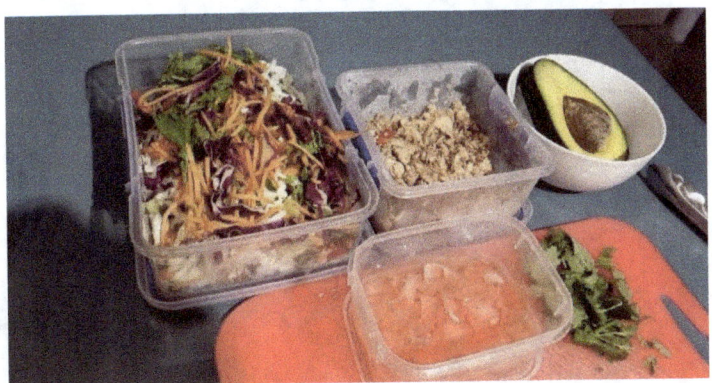

- 3 rice paper rounds
- 150g Paramount PINK salmon, drained
- Balsamic vinegar
- ½ avocado
- Pandaroo Sushi Ginger
- Fresh red chilli, chopped
- Coleslaw veg, dry
- Kaleslaw, with dressing
- Fresh coriander

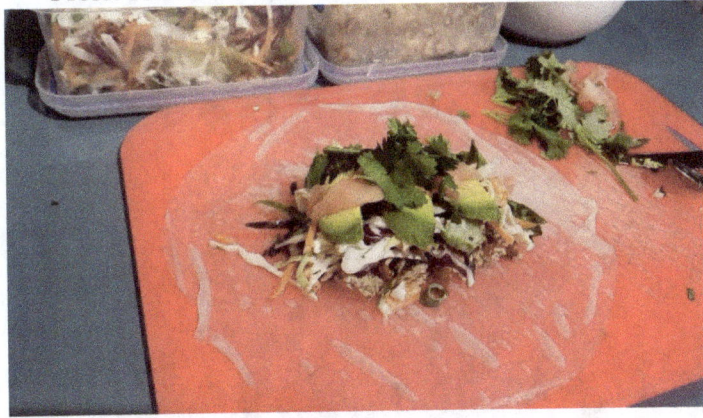

112. Pink salmon, nori, alfalfa, avo

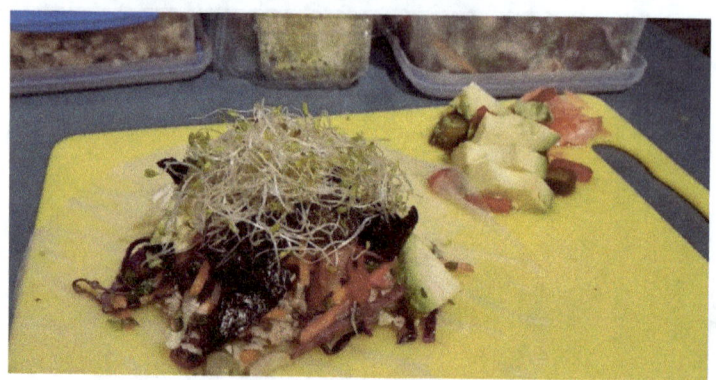

- 3 rice paper rounds
- 150g Paramount PINK salmon, drained
- Balsamic vinegar
- ½ avocado
- Pandaroo Sushi Ginger
- Pickled jalapenos, chopped
- Pickled red chilli, chopped
- Mixed coleslaw/kaleslaw
- Nori strips
- Alfalfa sprouts
- Poonsin Vietnamese spring roll dipping sauce

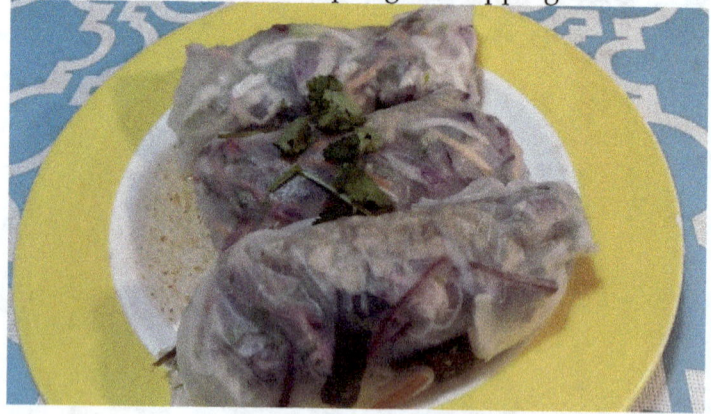

113. Pink salmon, coriander, lettuce

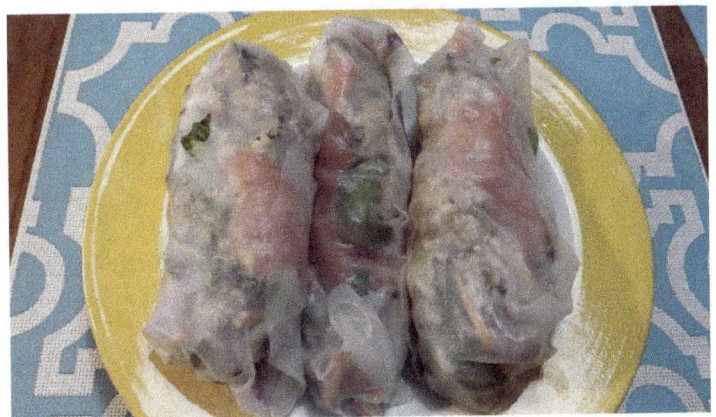

- 3 rice paper rounds
- 150g John West PINK salmon, drained
- Pandaroo Sushi Ginger
- Crunchy Coleslaw
- Iceberg lettuce
- Fresh coriander
- Poonsin Vietnamese Spring Roll Dipping Sauce

114. Pink salmon, avo, jalapenos, lime

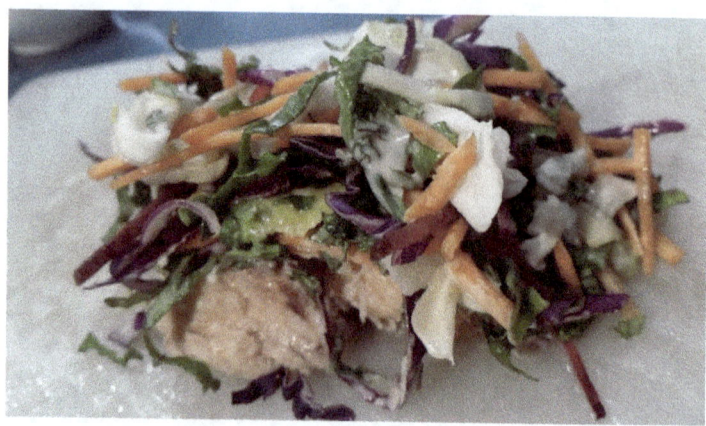

- 3 rice paper rounds
- 150g John West PINK salmon, drained
- ½ avocado
- Pickled jalapenos, chopped
- Lime juice
- Mixed coleslaw/kaleslaw, with dressing

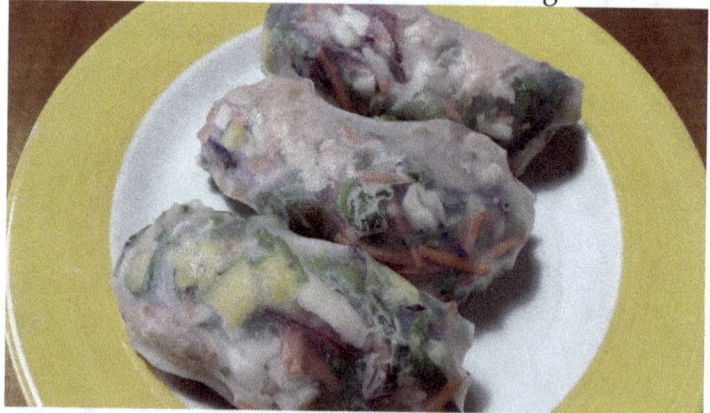

115. Pink salmon, olives, basil, balsamic

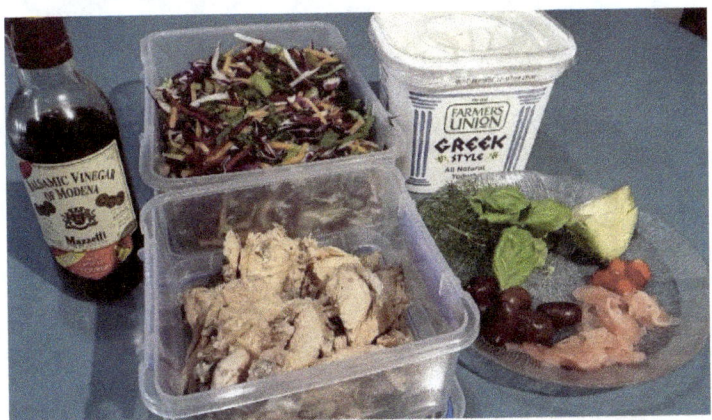

- 3 rice paper rounds
- 150g John West PINK salmon, drained
- Greek yoghurt
- ¼ avocado
- Balsamic vinegar
- Pandaroo Sushi Ginger
- Pickled red chilli, chopped
- 6 black olives, pitted and chopped
- Mixed coleslaw/kaleslaw
- Fresh herbs (Basil, fennel)

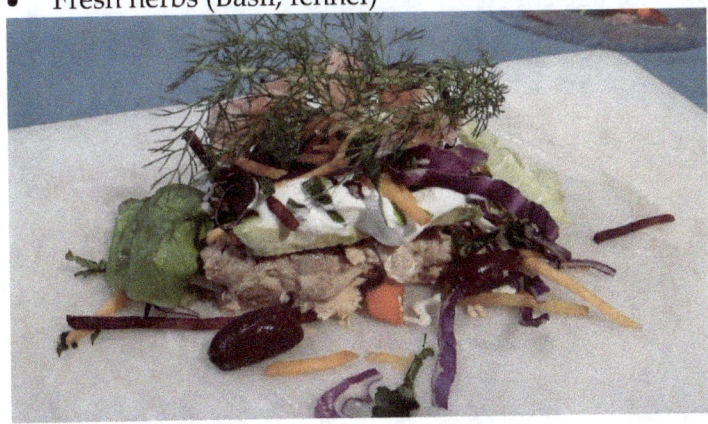

116. Pink salmon, Italian perfecto

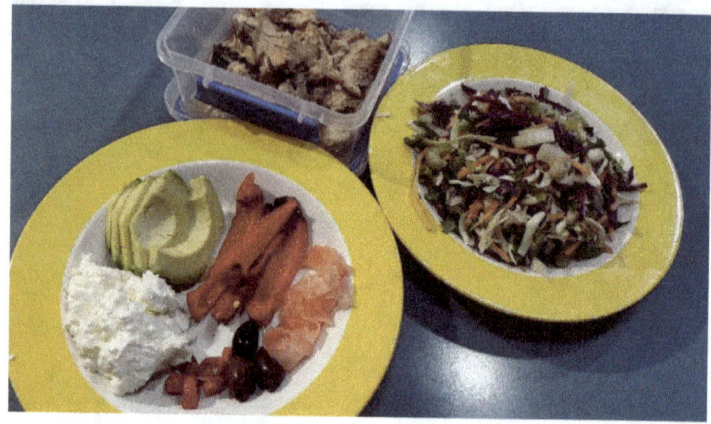

- 3 rice paper rounds
- 150g John West PINK salmon, drained
- ½ avocado
- Balsamic vinegar
- Pandaroo Sushi Ginger
- Pickled red chilli, chopped
- 6 black olives, pitted and chopped
- Roasted red capsicum, sliced
- Mixed coleslaw/kaleslaw
- Cottage cheese

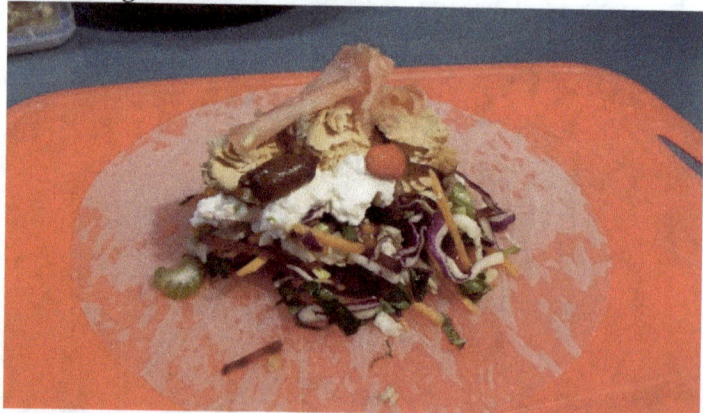

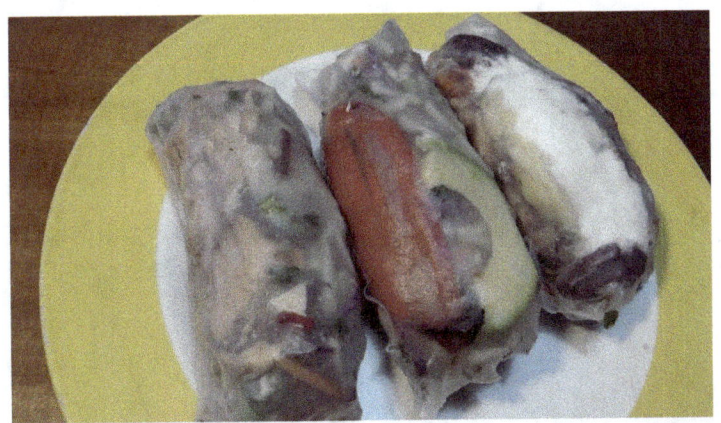

117. Pink salmon, guacamole

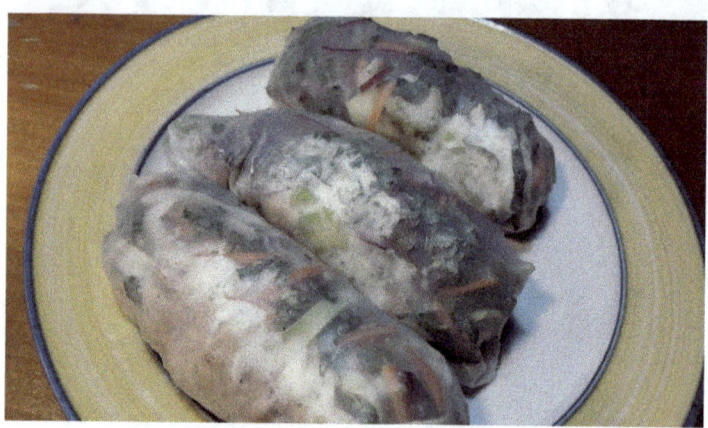

- 3 rice paper rounds
- 150g John West PINK salmon, drained
- To make GUACAMOLE – mix together,
    - Greek yoghurt
    - ¼ avocado
    - Teaspoon Conimex Sambal Oelek
    - Pickled jalapenos, chopped
    - Squeeze of fresh lime or lemon juice
- Mixed coleslaw/kaleslaw
- Lettuce

118. Pink and smoked salmon, Chang's

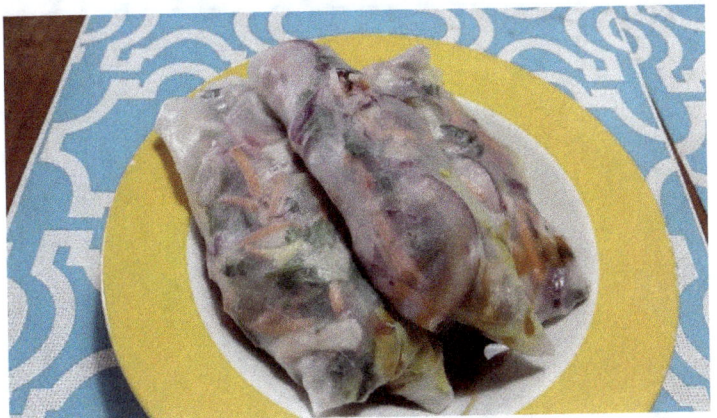

- 3 rice paper rounds
- 150g John West PINK salmon, drained
- 50g smoked salmon
- Pandaroo Sushi Ginger
- Pickled jalapenos, sliced
- Coleslaw
- Lettuce
- Chang's Fried Noodle Dipping Sauce

119. Pink salmon, jalapenos, mizuna

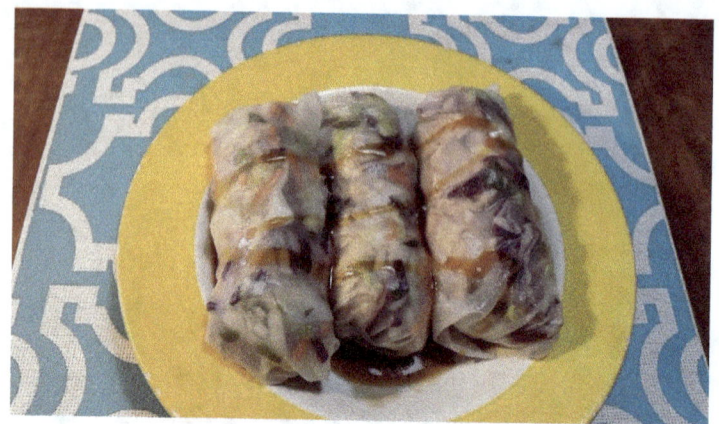

- 3 rice paper rounds
- 150g John West PINK salmon, drained
- Pandaroo Sushi Ginger
- Pickled jalapenos, sliced
- Lemon juice
- Thai mizuna salad kit, with Thai dressing

120. Layered PINK salmon stir-fry

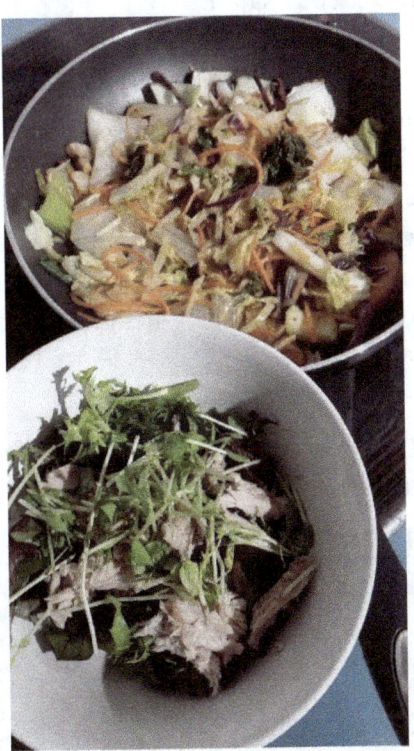

COOKING
In a large frypan, on high heat, add
- Teaspoon of Tom Yum paste
- ¼ cup water
- ½ tomato, chopped
- One large Swiss Brown mushroom, thinly sliced
- Splash of lime juice

Stir, then allow to cook for a couple of minutes.
Then add other vegetables.
- ½ baby bok choy, chopped
- Cup of wombok, chopped
- Cup of mixed coleslaw/Asian slaw

Cover with a lid until vegetables are wilted.

SERVING

In a bowl, construct your salad:
- Add a cup of mesculin mixed salad leaves, roughly chopped
- 200g tinned pink salmon, drained
- Chopped stems of Asian pea shoots (optional)
- Add the contents of the frypan on top of the salmon
- Add chopped shallots, coriander, and pea sprouts
- Add ¼ avocado, sliced
- Sprinkle with half a small packet of crispy fried shallots on top, and serve.

HINT: By layering the bowl with the hot veg on top of the salmon and salad greens, just enough heat will be transferred to the salmon and salad. No need to cook or heat separately.

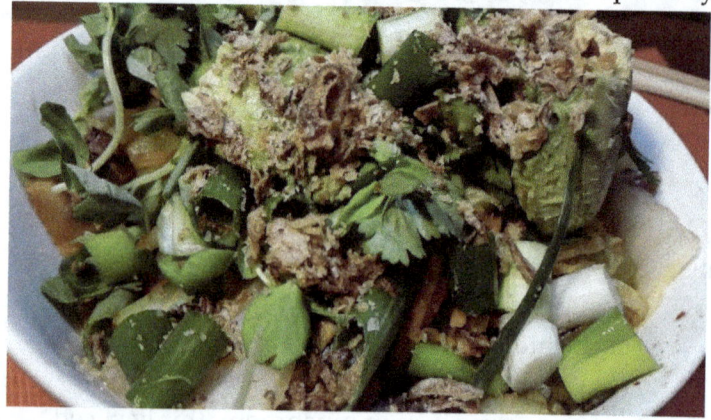

TINNED RED SALMON

Tinned RED SALMON is WILD CAUGHT, making it a healthier option than farmed salmon fillets. Being wild caught, tinned red salmon is free of all the chemical additives and artificial colouring fed to farmed fish.

Yes, RED SALMON is delicious, but it is expensive compared to tuna or pink salmon.

Yes, RED SALMON is high in omega-3s, but that is why it contains more calories per 100g than its cheaper cousins.

Nevertheless, I do love the flavour and texture of RED SALMON, so I treat myself about once a month. And because red salmon is so delicious straight from the can, you don't need to add vinegar or any other strong flavours when making your rice paper rolls. Keep it simple and fresh so the taste of the red salmon isn't buried under other flavours.

121. Red salmon, kaleslaw, jalapenos

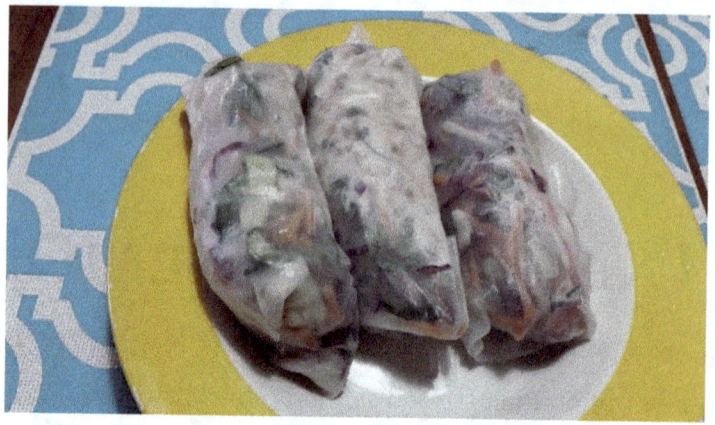

- 3 rice paper rounds
- 150g John West RED salmon, drained
- Greek yoghurt
- Pandaroo Sushi Ginger
- Pickled jalapenos, sliced
- Mixed kaleslaw/coleslaw

122. Red salmon, crunchy salad, ginger

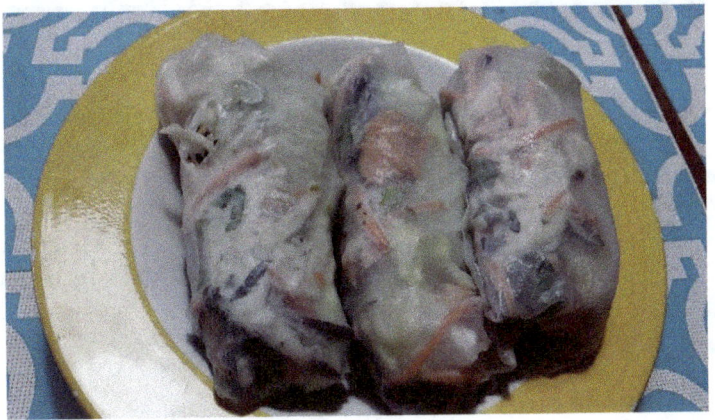

- 3 rice paper rounds
- 150g John West RED salmon, drained
- Pandaroo Sushi Ginger
- Iceberg lettuce
- Crunchy Coleslaw (with onion slices), dry
- Ranch dressing

123. Red salmon, jalapenos, sesame oil

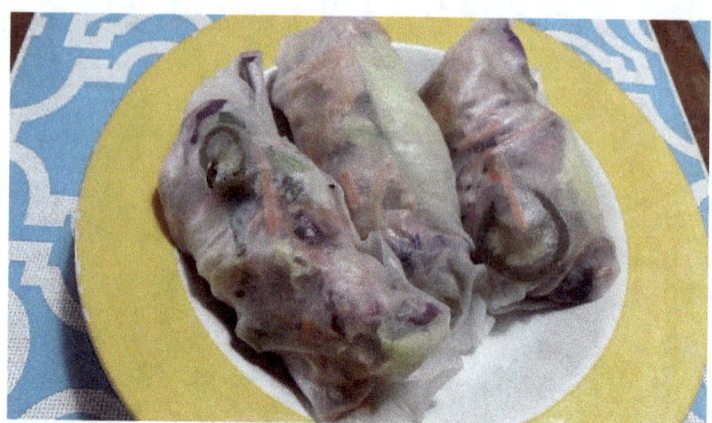

- 3 rice paper rounds
- 150g John West RED salmon, drained
- Greek yoghurt
- Pandaroo Sushi Ginger
- Pickled jalapenos, sliced
- Teaspoon of Balsamic vinegar
- A few drips of sesame oil
- Coleslaw
- Iceberg lettuce
- Poonsin Vietnamese Spring Roll Dipping Sauce

124. Red salmon, Italian bruschetta

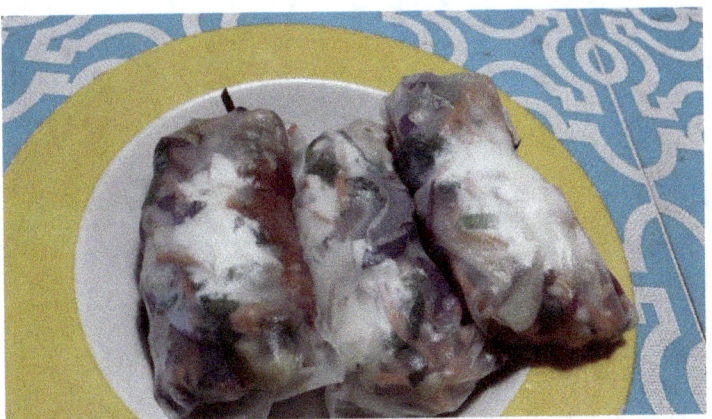

- 3 rice paper rounds
- 150g John West RED salmon, drained
- Greek yoghurt
- Bruschetta mix – chop or blend together
    - ½ fresh tomato
    - ½ red onion
    - Sprig of fresh basil
- 6 x black olives, pitted and sliced
- Mixed kaleslaw/coleslaw

125. Red salmon, ginger, kaleslaw

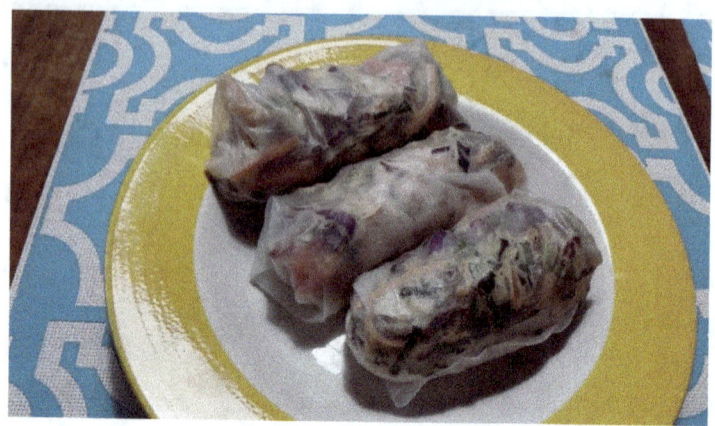

- 3 rice paper rounds
- 150g John West RED salmon, drained
- Greek yoghurt
- Pandaroo Sushi Ginger
- Pickled jalapenos, sliced
- Mixed kaleslaw/coleslaw/Southern slaw

126. Red salmon, cos lettuce, alfalfa

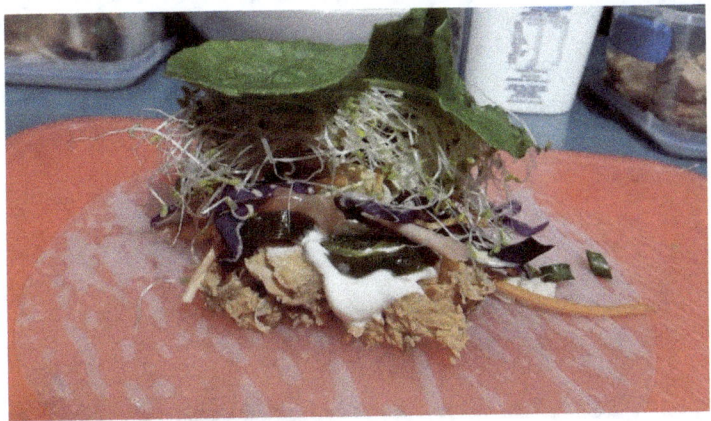

- 3 rice paper rounds
- 150g John West RED salmon, drained
- Greek yoghurt
- Pandaroo Sushi Ginger
- Pickled jalapenos, sliced
- Southern Style coleslaw kit, with dressing
- Baby cos lettuce
- Alfalfa sprouts

127. Red salmon, avo, alfalfa, Caesar

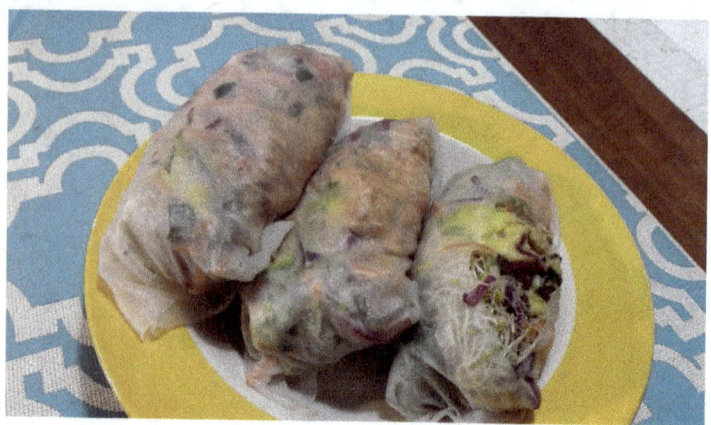

- 3 rice paper rounds
- 150g John West RED salmon, drained
- Greek yoghurt
- ¼ avocado
- Pandaroo Sushi Ginger
- Fresh green chilli, chopped
- Kaleslaw
- Baby cos lettuce
- Alfalfa sprouts
- Caesar dressing

128. Red salmon, hot chilli, shallots

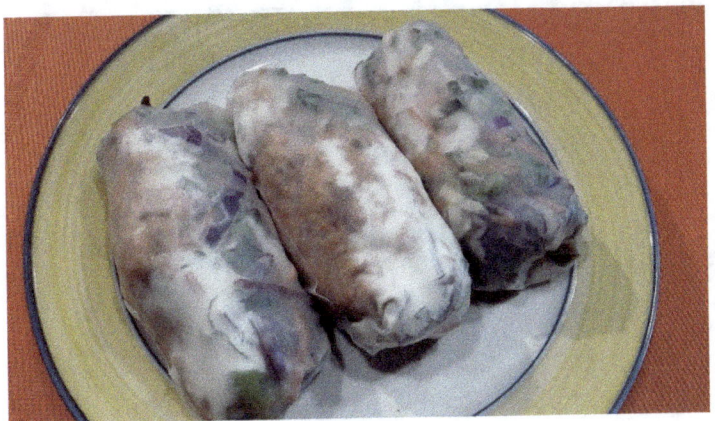

- 3 rice paper rounds
- 150g John West RED salmon, drained
- Greek yoghurt
- ¼ avocado
- Pandaroo Sushi Ginger
- Fresh shallots, chopped
- Trident hot chilli sauce
- Mixed kaleslaw/coleslaw

129. Red salmon, avo, vinegar, herbs

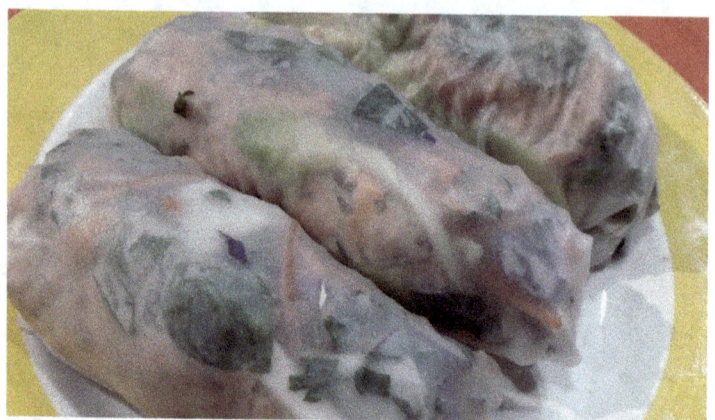

- 3 rice paper rounds
- 150g John West RED salmon, drained
- Greek yoghurt
- ¼ avocado
- Fresh red chilli, chopped
- Drizzle of white salad vinegar over salmon
- Mixed kaleslaw/Thai mizuna salad kit
- Asian herbs (Vietnamese mint, Thai basil)

130. Spicy red salmon salad bowl

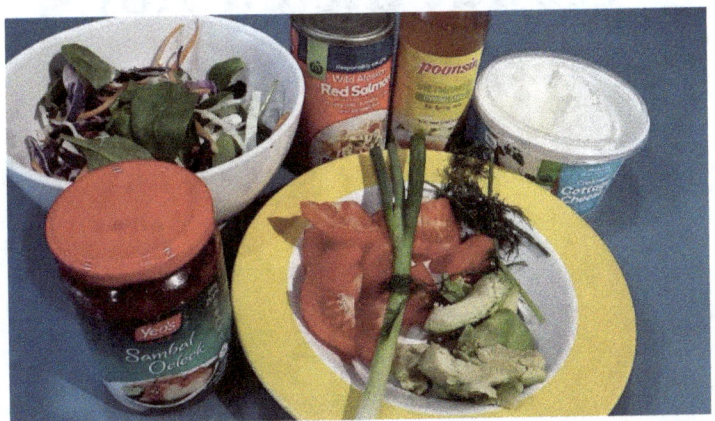

- 3 rice paper rounds
- 150g John West RED salmon, drained
- ½ avocado
- 1 x fresh ripe tomato, sliced
- 1 x shallot, diced
- Sambal Oelek
- Mixed coleslaw/Thai mizuna salad kit
- Cottage cheese
- Fresh dill
- Poonsin Vietnamese Spring Roll Dipping Sauce

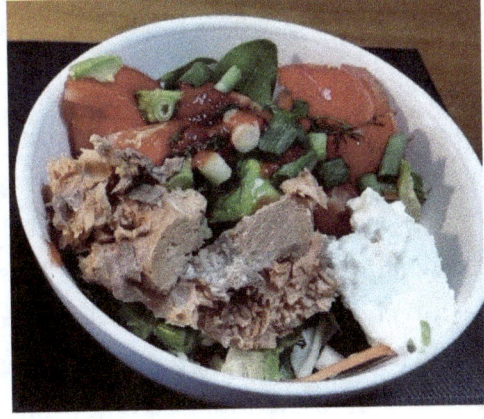

About the author

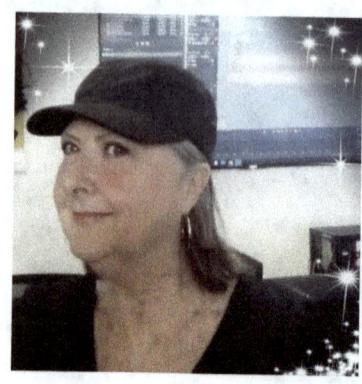

Kathryn M. James

MASR(Health), BScBiomedical(Hons), GDipA(Coun), GDipFDRP

Kathryn M. James is an award-winning Australian author. The primary book in this series, **THE HUNGER HERO DIET©: How to Lose Weight and Break the Depression Cycle – Without Exercise, Drugs or Surgery**, was the culmination of 10 years of multi-disciplinary studies in the health sciences, combined with the lived experience of depression-related obesity.

The companion set of cookbooks in the FAST AND EASY RECIPES series provides additional resources for anyone wanting to eat better, feel better, and lose weight.

These recipes show how eating well can be FAST AND EASY, with a few simple ingredients you can be swap in and out to suit. Each recipe is for ONE single serve, so you never have to cook huge amounts of food, unless you want to.

Website: https://KMJamesWriter.com/
Email: KMJamesWriter@outlook.com

Titles in the HUNGER HERO DIET series

THE HUNGER HERO DIET: How to Lose Weight and Break the Depression Cycle – Without Exercise, Drugs or Surgery
ISBN 978-0-6455255-0-2   ebook
ISBN 978-0-6455255-1-9   paperback print book
ISBN 978-0-6455255-2-6   hardcover print book

The HUNGER HERO DIET – Fast and Easy Recipe Series #1: Cooking with FISH
ISBN 978-0-6455255-5-7   ebook
ISBN 978-0-6455255-3-3   paperback print book

The HUNGER HERO DIET – Fast and Easy Recipe Series #2: PRAWNS and OTHER SEAFOOD
ISBN 978-0-6455255-6-4   ebook
ISBN 978-0-6455255-4-0   paperback print book

The HUNGER HERO DIET – Fast and Easy Recipe Series #3: Tinned FISH Vietnamese-style
ISBN 978-0-6455255-7-1   ebook
ISBN 978-0-6455255-8-8   paperback print book

www.ingramcontent.com/pod-product-compliance
Lightning Source LLC
Chambersburg PA
CBHW050313010526
44107CB00055B/2230